All of Me

To Geoff
lots of love
Andrée xxx

Andrée Dignon

All of Me

A Fuller Picture of Anorexia

PETER LANG
Oxford · Bern · Berlin · Bruxelles · Frankfurt am Main · New York · Wien

Bibliographic information published by Die Deutsche Bibliothek
Die Deutsche Bibliothek lists this publication in the Deutsche Nationalbibliografie; detailed bibliographic data is available on the Internet at ‹http://dnb.ddb.de›.

British Library and Library of Congress Cataloguing-in-Publication Data:
A catalogue record for this book is available from The British Library, Great Britain, and from The Library of Congress, USA

Cover Image: Melancholy Girl by Brenda York. 2007.
ISBN 978-3-03911-075-9

Hochfeldstrasse 32, Postfach 746, CH-3000 Bern 9, Switzerland
info@peterlang.com, www.peterlang.com, www.peterlang.net

Printed in Germany

To Neil with love

Contents

Acknowledgements

I have some heartfelt thanks to convey to those people who have helped make this book possible. First of all, my sincere thanks go to Dr. Ellen Annandale and Dr. Jane Pilcher of Leicester University. Their informed and intelligent suggestions were invaluable in rendering this book in its current form. Secondly, I send warm thanks to the specialist registrar who interviewed the anorexic patients, both for her tireless work in conducting the interviews and for her generosity in allowing her work to be subject to critical scrutiny. Such self-reflection shows a true commitment to advancing the boundaries of research. My thanks also go to the director of the eating disorders unit in which the study was based, for allowing the study access to his patients. In addition, I thank Becky Congdon, from the University of Coventry, for all her technical support.

In particular I want to thank the patients themselves. Their candid, honest and open testimony has formed the empirical backbone to this study. In sharing their insight into their disorder their contribution has been invalulable.

Most of all, I thank my partner, Neil Hanney. Without Neil's kindness, love and support this book would not have been possible.

Chapter 1
The Story of the Anorexic Stereotype

Introduction

This book is a study of anorexia. It describes an investigation conducted in an eating disorders unit in England between 1985 and 2001. During this time, information was gathered from 104 anorexics. These patients talked about their illness and what they felt had caused it. They described their social origins and educational background and ultimately provided a wealth of information. This information forms the basis of this book.

The data gathered was used in two ways. Firstly it was used to tell us something about the experience of anorexics themselves. The detailed accounts provided by these patients provided a window into the life of the anorexic. Secondly however (and for the purpose of this book, perhaps more importantly) the information was used as a yardstick against which to measure the interpretations which doctors place on the disorder. The book therefore asks whether clinical constructions of anorexia always reflect patients' experiences.

The book therefore examines a highly specific area of anorexia – the clinical knowledge that surrounds the illness. I argue that medicine has constructed a 'stereotype' of the anorexic, as young, bright and middle class. According to this stereotype, this bright, affluent, youngster becomes anorexic because she is afraid of fatness and afraid to grow up.

A stereotype may be viewed as a construct that applies a specific identity to the stereotyped group (Pickering, 2001, Hinton, 2000, MacCrae et al, 1996, Leyens et al 1994). This identity is based on a single specific characteristic (Hinton, 2000:7). This single characteristic may be a broad category, such as race or gender, or it may be more specific such as being 'a blonde', or 'an anorexic' or 'an accountant' or 'a redhead'. The corollary of being defined according to this characteristic is that a range of additional pre-defined traits are attributed to members of this group (Pickering, 2001). Blondes, for example, are 'dumb', while accountants are 'dull' and 'redheads' are 'fiery'. This book argues that the category 'anorexia' constitutes a stereotype, where pre-defined traits, such as youth, affluence and maturity fear, are attributed to anorexic patients.

The stereotype of the anorexic has developed over many years. This chapter identifies the historical development of the concept of anorexia and explains changes in this concept by referring to the sociology of knowledge. The chapter then argues that clinicians usually search for 'certainty' in making diagnoses and that this certainty may give rise to stereotypical definitions of the disorder. These definitions, the chapter explains, will be analysed in the book using sociological theory. At the outset in this chapter, a definition of sociological theory in the area of knowledge will be supplied.

The Sociology of Knowledge

The sociology of knowledge argues that science is 'socially produced' (Berger and Luckmann, 1966, Thrift, 1994, Burke 2000). Forms of knowledge (including medical knowledge) develop out of the social milieu of which they are part (Berger and Luckmann, 1966, Thrift, 1994). In the clinical milieu, a 'positivist' approach to knowledge is adopted, where the methods of natural science are privileged. As a result, clinicians may search for scientific certainty even when diagnosing complex illnesses such as anorexia.

Such complex illnesses are defined using 'knowledge', developed by psychiatrists. This knowledge is 'treated as universal truth, although it is evident to any outsider that it [...] take[s] its character [...] from the habits of the life of the group' (Veblen, 1906, quoted in Burke, 2000:4). Such a group can define and validate what is accepted as knowledge (Bourdieu, 1996). As Foucault (1986), explains, knowledge takes a particular form as a result of discourse and negotiation. Interpretations are given to specific behaviour (such as self-starvation) by powerful groups (such as clinicians). In this way certain constructions of knowledge develop while others do not. Clinical knowledge therefore, 'is made up of doctrines which themselves demand evaluation.' (Barnes, 1982, quoted in Thrift, 1994:397).

Physicians, however, may espouse their doctrines with certainty. The doctor's commitment to establishing clinical 'facts' may lead him or her to look for certainty where none exists. This search for certainty has been explored in the sociology of science (Collins and Pinch, 1994, Elston, 1997, Woolgar, 1988). The sociology of science focuses specifically on 'scientific' knowledge and argues that even in 'hard' science, social processes (such as selective funding) influence knowledge production. This renders science less neutral than might be supposed. Scholarship from the sociology of science will thus be referred to in this chapter.

This book will contend that forms of knowledge can be as much the product of the social world as they are manifestations of objective phenomenon. 'When one inhabits a system', however, 'it generally looks like common sense. Only by comparison can one see it as one system among others' (Burke, 2000:2). An interesting method of comparing different systems is by tracing the historical evolution of particular concepts, and by comparing the ways these concepts have been defined over time. The central concept in this book is the entity of 'anorexia'. A discussion of the historical development of the diagnosis of anorexia will now be offered.

The Historical Development of the Diagnosis of Anorexia

Anorexia, as currently understood, was defined over a period of many years. Early cases of 'holy anorexia' from the thirteenth to the seventeenth centuries, were interpreted in religious terms. In the eighteenth and nineteenth centuries more 'modern' accounts of self-starvation began to emerge. The formation of the disorder can thus be traced over five historical periods:

'Holy anorexia' and self-starvation prior to 1874
1874–1918: Gull's 'discovery' of anorexia nervosa
1918–1945: The somatic approach to anorexia
1945–1970s: The re-emergence of psychology
1970s onwards: 'Certainty' in a multi-disciplinary context

'Holy anorexia' and self-starvation prior to 1874

Prior to 1874, fasting was considered to be performed largely for religious reasons. Early cases of self-starvation, dating from the thirteenth century, are attributed to 'holy anorexia' (Brumberg, 1988a) practised by female ascetics. Mary of Oignes, Beatrice of Nazareth and Catherine of Sienna all subsisted on the barest intake of seeds, herbs and water. As a result, Catherine of Sienna starved herself to death (Tolstrupp, 1990). Her suicide, however, was interpreted very differently to the behaviour of today's anorexics. The biological processes which led to Catherine's death were identical to the experience of the modern anorexic. But at a social level, the experience was entirely different. Catherine died a revered and honoured saint. Modern anorexics are viewed as the victims of a tragic medical illness, brought on by abuse, unhappiness and neglect (Palmer et al, 1990, Tolstrupp, 1990).

In the mediaeval period, the self-starvation of holy anorexics was not seen as a medical problem. True, these ascetics suffered the (sometimes fatal) physiological effects of malnutrition, but such privation was viewed as religious, and was therefore left untreated. Self-starvation was a noble activity, beneficial to the whole of humankind as a sacrifice to atone for human sin. Ascetics were often of a higher social status than healers, and were thus allowed to continue their activities uninterrupted (Porter, 2002). Indeed, it would have been viewed as sacrilegious for healers to have meddled with the ascetic's noble calling.

This tolerance may be attributed to the acceptance of 'holy' insanity. 'The church entertained [that starving] ascetics might be possessed by a good madness' (Porter, 2002:19) which added to the store of saintly virtue and helped to assuage people's sins. Nevertheless, madness in the middle ages was normally viewed with horror. Insanity was understood as the work of the devil, often punishable by execution. This 'fundamentalist' attitude however was largely abandoned in the seventeenth century. After the English civil war (1642–1651), religious extremism began to be rejected (Porter, 2002) and 'doctors replaced the clergy in handling the insane' (Porter, 2002:33). Enlightenment thinkers of the late seventeenth and eighteenth centuries thus began to use medical explanations to describe mental illness.

Such a view was reflected in the progressive and systematic approach of many physicians, including those charged with managing the starving. Pinel (1745–1826) and Esquirol (1772–1840) for example, focussed on illness course (rather than symptom intensity) (Porter, 2002). It thus became social practice to observe starving patients, record case histories and publicise findings. During this period, diseases began to be scientifically classified (a process often attributed to Thomas Sydenham (1624–1698) (Sigerist, 1933)). Rather than using general labels such as 'ague' or 'pox', distinct disease entities such as 'scarlet fever', began to be identified.

Disease classification was a progressive development in the history of medicine. It allowed syndromes to be isolated and studied, and it pre-empted later public health and epidemiological measures (used to tackle disorders such as cholera (Jones, 1991)). At the same time however, the movement to classify disorders, including self-starvation, helped to distance the concept of an illness from the patient who was suffering from it. By giving illnesses their own unique identities, it was often the disease that was the focus of interest rather than the patients themselves. The relationship between the patient and the doctor was thus altered by the emergence of 'scientific medicine' (Hepworth, 1999, Armstrong, 1982, Jewson, 1976)

Society's construction of appetite loss in the early nineteenth century reflected these social processes. Self-starvation began to be defined as a medical problem, reflecting the shifting social influence of science over religion as a dominant paradigm (Porter, 2002). As a medical problem, self-starvation could 'be resolved by a set of predictable empirical validation techniques, around the clock watches, calculations of food intake, observation and measurement of excrement and weighing of the body' (Brumberg, 1988a:57). Appetite loss however, tended to be lumped together with other 'wasting' diseases such as tuberculosis (Tolstrupp, 1990). Reports of anorexia were patchy (Tolstrupp, 1990) and even where a 'tentative' anorexic diagnosis was appropriate, few such diagnoses were made (Parry-Jones, 1985). From the mediaeval to the Victorian period, therefore, food refusal was explained either in physiological or religious terms. In 1874, for the first time 'anorexia' was described as a mental illness.

1874–1918: Gulls 'discovery' of anorexia nervosa

In 1874 the term 'anorexia nervosa' was coined by William Gull (Palmer, 1989). A year earlier the term 'anorexia hysterique' had been coined by the French physician Laségue (Hepworth, 1999, Russell, 2000). Though Gull and Laségue differed in respect of the emphasis they placed on hysteria as a component of the diagnosis, both emphasised the psychological aspects of the disorder (Parry-Jones, 1985). Shortly after Gull and Laségue's 'identification' of anorexia, several reports of the illness (Brumberg, 1988a) began to appear in medical literature (Parry-Jones, 1985). Many of these papers recommended therapy based on Gull and Laségue's suggestions. This resembled a modern approach and consisted of regular observation and meals and removing the patient from her family. 'The secret of success in treating the case was in removing the patient from her home, putting her under a good nurse, and using tact, encouragement, food and good morale, with very little medicine' (Lloyd, 1893:276 cited in Vanderycken and Lowenkopf, 1990:534). Between 1874–1918, therefore, the condition of anorexia was publicly identified and labeled. This interest in anorexia however, began to wane after the turn of the century. At this time, Gull and Laségue's psychological focus was replaced by a physiological or somatic emphasis. This somatic approach will now be discussed.

1918–1945 The somatic approach to anorexia

After 1918, cases of anorexia were explained physiologically (Tolstrupp, 1990). The reasons for this are unclear. However, in the 1920s and 1930s there was a general resurgence in organic explanations for all forms of mental illness (Hepworth, 1999), of which anorexia was a rare (and, at the time, an 'insignificant') example. As such it was subjected to the same social processes as other kinds of mental disorder. After 1918, extreme physical therapies (such as lobotomy) were used to treat insanity (Porter, 2002), and anorexics occasionally received such treatment (Hepworth, 1999). In the 20s, 30s and early 40s anorexia was thus regarded as a physical disturbance (sometimes referred to as 'Simmonds' disease, (Parry-Jones, 1985:96)). In the late 30s and 40s, however, Ryle (1936), Sheldon (1939) and Sheehan and Summers (1949) slowly reestablished an interest in the psychology of anorexia. The next section describes the manner in which during the post-war period, psychological interpretations of anorexia re-emerged.

1945–1970s The re-emergence of psychology

Having occupied a secondary place in medical knowledge, the diagnosis of anorexia once more gained the physician's attention in the 1940s (Sheldon, 1939, Sheehan and Summers, 1949, Tolstrupp, 1990). A post war shift in emphasis from the study of schizophrenia to the study of neuroses heralded a new emphasis on the importance of psychology and observation in the management of psychiatric illness (Sheldon, 1939, Habermas, 1991). Such an emphasis echoed Gull and Laségue's approach of the late nineteenth century. In Habermas's view (1991), the 're-discovery' of anorexia was largely due to the work of a single psychiatrist, Ludwig Binswanger (1881–1966). In describing the case of Ellen West, Binswanger's 'professional training enabled him [...] to almost re-discover anorexia by himself' (Habermas, 1991:361). By systematically observing her alimentary behaviour, Binswanger was persuaded that Ellen West's case was indeed anorexia nervosa.

1970s onwards: 'certainty' in a multi disciplinary context

At the same time as anorexia was rediscovered by Binswanger, there was also an explosive growth in 'objective' rating instruments (Wing, 1980) used to measure eating disorder. This reflected a general trend in psychiatry whereby objective rating scales were increasingly applied. These scales measured symptoms using closed-ended, validated questionnaires. A number of 'objective' anorexia scales were developed in the 1970s (Garner and Garfinkel, 1979, Garner et al, 1983b), largely based on criteria such as 'weight phobia', (APA 1994). The social valuation of 'hard' science at this time thus led psychiatrists to attribute highly 'certain' criteria to the disorder.

This search for certainty however belied the rich debate surrounding anorexia. Theories of anorexia began to proliferate in the 1970s including Bruch's (1978), and Crisp's (1995) paradigms, based on family theory. Anorexics were described as coming from isolated, uncommunicative and 'enmeshed' families, where mothers had failed to instill self-sufficiency and independence in their daughters. Anorexia was thus theorised as a flight from full social and sexual maturity, largely as a result of poor mothering. Such mother blaming reflected what was occurring in psychiatry generally, where mothers were routinely identified as the source of mental disorder (Caplan, 1990, Mackler, 1976, Grolnick and Gurland, 2002, Wedenoja, 1991, Ruskay-Rabinor, 1994).

Some opposition to this mother blaming approach was evident however in the work of feminists, many of whom were highly critical of psychiatry's tendency to cite mothers as the cause of mental illness (Ruskay-Rabinor, 1994, Wedenoja, 1991). As well as critiquing mother blaming, feminists also emphasised the importance of society and women's position in it, in 'causing' anorexia (Orbach, 1993, Lawrence, 1995). Social institutions such as the beauty industry and the media were identified as damaging to women. Such institutions were also critiqued by psychiatrists (Garner et al, 1983a, Dolan et al, 1990). Multi-disciplinary explanations therefore predominated from the 1970s. These explanations and other 'historical' issues in the emergence of anorexia will now be analysed with reference to the sociology of knowledge.

Anorexia and the Sociology of Knowledge

As indicated above, the complex historical development of specific ways of viewing self-starvation may be analysed with reference to the sociology of knowledge (Kuhn, 1966, Mannheim, 1952, Elias, 1991). The development of anorexia as a diagnosis in its current form can be explained by developments in the state of knowledge at a given point in time. As Kuhn (1966) explains, ideas come into being, are modified by social processes and thus attain a particular form. 'Losing' theories disappear and are usually superseded by more 'refined' interpretations (Kuhn, 1966). Like Kuhn, Mannheim (1952) argues that knowledge thus 'excludes a large number of possible modes of thought [...] and [...] restricts expression [...] to certain circumscribed possibilities' (Mannheim, 1952:291). These 'circumscribed possibilities' come to dominate the manner in which a diagnosis such as anorexia is expressed. Specific interpretations of appetite loss (such as 'weight phobia' in the twentieth century) thus become privileged.

This process is not unilinear but complex (Mannheim, 1952). Specific theories compete, (for example competing somatic and psychological theories of anorexia in the 1930s), before one theory (the psychological) becomes dominant. 'There is scarcely a single intellectual position [...] which has not changed through history and which even in the present does not appear in many forms' (Mannheim, 1952:69). In the twentieth century, the knowledge of natural science was privileged (Mannheim, 1952). Such knowledge is based on positivism which aims to establish general laws. Even in the natural sciences however, knowledge is

> much more varied than textbook logic would have us believe [...] different modes of thought are characterized in the first place by [...] models and these models differ [...] We must [therefore] constantly ask ourselves how [...] a given type of social situation gives rise to a given interpretation'. (Mannheim, 1952:71–206)

It may be argued the 'social situation' of William Gull helped to give rise to his identification of anorexia. Prior to Gull's definition, religious interpretations of anorexia were beginning to be replaced with medical ones (Brumberg, 1988a). As a result of the enlightenment in the seventeenth, and eighteenth centuries a social context emerged which facilitated a shift from religious to rational explanations (Porter, 2002, Mannheim, 1952). It was in such a context that medicine became institutionalised as a profession. This culminated in the 1858 Medical (Registration) Act, which specified that only those legally or duly qualified (Witz, 1992:73) could practice medicine. By establishing itself as a profession medicine successfully established hegemony in defining illness in general and anorexia in particular. As an eminent physician working at this time (with access to patients, and the opportunity to publish his findings), Gull was ideally situated to 'discover' the illness of anorexia. Gulls definition may also be seen as a bid for prestigue, with Gull aiming in Hepworth's words to establish himself as a 'great [man] of science'.

Gull was thus in the right social context to identify anorexia in the nineteenth century. The social context in which recent ideas about anorexia have developed was described by Mizrachi in 2002. Mizrachi argues that, since 1957, the focus in defining anorexia became concentrated mainly on standardised bodily symptoms (such as amenorrhea). This was consistent with the 'power base' of medicine, which rested on the legitimate assessment of physical illness. Dissident, holistic, voices, Mizrachi explains, gradually became assimilated into the psychiatric mainstream. I argue in this book that this process of standardisation and medicalisation has continued and may have led to inaccuracy in the way anorexia is interpreted.

Mizrachi (and Mannheim) suggested that scientific theories change and develop over time. Like these researchers, Elias (1991) also emphasises the historical development of knowledge. Elias, however, stresses the centrality of language symbols. For Elias, the way in which knowledge is symbolically represented is central to the forms which knowledge acquires. 'There is nature there is culture, there is knowledge [...] and the all embracing symbols of language, but how they all cohere together is a question that is rarely asked' (Elias, 1991:89). Knowledge is therefore not 'a stationary object of the natural sciences' (1991:89), but develops over time by being symbolically produced through language. Since the entire social world which humans inhabit is symbolised through language, Elias rejected the belief that 'one fine day humans will wake up to find that they know the objects of knowledge independent of the fact that they are objects of human knowledge [themselves]' (1991:7). For Elias therefore, the scientist acquires knowledge as a social activity rather than as the result of their individual endeavours in isolation from the social world.

Elias was not alone in identifying that the acquisition of knowledge is a social process. Such an assertion was also made by Harding in 1991. She explains that the sciences are in 'every respect socially situated [they] are part and parcel [...] of the social order from which they emerge' (1991:11–37). As Harding and Elston (1997) explain, the development of technology (such as the microscope) moved the focus of medical investigation from the patient to the micro-organism. This, combined with social changes, (such as the legalisation of human dissection after the reformation), shifted the focus from the 'bedside' to the laboratory and the hospital (Jewson, 1976, Elston, 1997). Demand for bodies to dissect promoted a case study approach. This case study model was ultimately applied in the 'discovery' of anorexia. With the growth of scientific methodology it became possible to isolate the source of the illness, to standardise its diagnosis and to share this standardised interpretation with other clinicians. These processes of increased communication and competition between peers are evident in Gull and Laségue's uncovering of anorexia.

With the growth of standardisation and opportunities to share findings with peers, the health of populations became as important a focus as the health of individuals (Armstrong, 1995, 1982). This lead to the search for commonalties which in the case of anorexia eventually produced the anorexic stereotype. The demographic elements of the stereotype (for example the model of the anorexic as middle class) can be traced to this epidemiological focus, while cognitive elements (such as maturity fear) reflect sexist definitions of the sufferer as recalcitrant child refusing to grow up. It is also appropriate to ask why 'fat phobia' arose as a key symptom of anorexia in the psychiatric model at this point in time. Society currently constructs women as vain and obsessed with appearance. When they refuse to eat this must be because they do not want to get fat. Hence 'fat phobia' is a central element of the anorexic stereotype.

Constructions of 'femininity' are therefore central to anorexic knowledge. The theory of knowledge advanced by Elias however lacked any specific commentary on the position of women. Elias's early work was published in the 1950s and 1960s (when women's second class status was taken for granted), and this may in part explain women's 'invisibility' in his early research. His latest publication, however, first appeared in 1991, long after women's experiences had begun to be integrated into mainstream sociology. Even at this time, Elias had little to say about knowledge in relation to women. Hepworth (1999), however addresses this shortfall by taking a feminist approach to the development of 'anorexia'. Drawing on feminist and post-structuralist writing, Hepworth explains how anorexia was finally 'recognised'. Prevailing knowledge about women's disease in the nineteenth century was 'profoundly ideological' (1999: 28) and was used to construct women, particularly young women, as irrational and prone to conditions such as anorexia. Though Gull and Laségue's recommendations for therapy were comparatively progressive they continued to construct women as deficient and in need of supervision. Also, the treatment given to anorexics at the time reflected an attempt to control these women, who found themselves 'managed in a medical domain' (1999:35).

Hepworth analysed these developments from a woman centred perspective. Other feminists have joined her in this enterprise. Such scholars have argued that science 'legimitates womens inferiority' (Elston, 1997:25) and constructs knowledge from the male point of view (Oakley, 1992, Webb, 1993, Belenky et al, 1986). People, feminists argue, have different standpoints depending on the gender to which they belong. 'Knowledge' is constructed from the standpoint of the male, a process that is exemplified in the construction of medical knowledge. Martin, for example (1987) describes the 'value-laden' descriptions of male and female reproductive organs in clinical textbooks. The penis and spermatozoa are described using positive words such as 'remarkable', while the menses are described using negative words such as 'debris'. Such gender bias may lead to the rendering of normal female experience, such as menstruation and childbirth, as illnesses (Martin, 1987, Oakley, 1987, Stanworth, 1987). This process is known as 'medicalisation' (Higgs, 2003), and is clearly evident in the diagnosis of psychiatric illness, (Kutchins and Kirk, 1997, Szasz, 1976, Young, 1992), including anorexia. Such illnesses may be a justifiable 'anger response' to the conditions of women's lives, but are nevertheless constructed solely as maladies. One therefore wonders whether women are actually ill or 'merely diagnosed a such because of the discourse associating femininity and psychological infirmity' (Ussher, 1991:164).

This gender bias underpins the focus of many research studies, as well as influencing the subjects selected and the generation of data and theory (Harding, 1991). 'Whoever gets to define what counts as a scientific problem also gets a powerful role in shaping the picture of the world that results from scientific research' (Harding, 1991:70). Male 'experts' have thus identified women as a 'problem' (Ehrenreich and English, 1989) and have appealed to science to legitimate sexist interpretations of 'women's' disorders. As a result 'truth itself has become genderized' (Fox-Keller, 1985:87). As this 'unconscious mythology' is recognised however it is possible for science 'not to be bound by such mythology' (Fox-Keller, 1985:93).

The feminist work produced by Harding, Ehrenreich and English has therefore highlighted the sexism inherent in psychiatric knowledge. In so doing, this work represents an advance over the work of Elias. Like Elias however, feminists identify the development of science, (and in particular psychiatric diagnoses) as a social phenomenon. This process has involved standardising the criteria applied to diagnoses such as anorexia. The social development of standardised psychiatric diagnoses will now be discussed.

The Social Development of Standardised Psychiatric Diagnoses

The search for certainty in psychiatric diagnoses

Anorexia is currently constructed as a disorder of uncertain cause (Palmer, 1989). My argument has so far proposed that the theories that attempt to explain it have changed and evolved over time (Lee, 1996). In the 1970s for example, fear of maturity and social class were considered important (Bruch, 1978, Crisp et al, 1976) while in the 1980s the effect of adverse life events (Palmer et al, 1990) and the use of anorexia as a strategy of control (Lawrence, 1984) were stressed. Similarly, the rules for making a clinical diagnosis of anorexia have been periodically revised by the clinical community. Today 15 per cent of body weight must be shed for the diagnosis to be made, whereas in the 1980s, a reduction of one quarter was required (Lee, 1996). Currently accepted explanations, therefore represent today's 'best buy' (Palmer, 1989:2), and will eventually be superseded by new interpretations.

The category 'anorexia nervosa' is therefore fluid and negotiable, and the criteria applied to the diagnosis may be contested and changed. In the construction of clinical knowledge, the process of modifying diagnostic criteria however, tends to take the form whereby old 'certainties' are removed and substituted by new 'certainties' (Kutchins and Kirk, 1997). This process of scientific standardisation and legitimacy has played a pivotal role in the construction of psychiatric diagnoses. The development of validated criteria began in the 19th century (Fisher, 2001, Witz, 1992, Freidson, 1970a) and was one of the key mechanisms through which medicine acquired public trust and acknowledgement. From the perspective of the psychiatric community, this process of 'validating' diagnostic rules also had the advantage of making psychiatric criteria more 'scientific', thus improving psychiatry's standing in relation to other more physiological clinical specialisms (Mizrachi, 2002). The mechanisms by which anorexic criteria became progressively more 'objective' and 'scientific' are described by Mizrachi as follows:

> [From the 1940s onwards] the growing number of competing […] non-medical approaches to anorexia had minimal effect on the hard core somatic medicine that continued to focus its attention on the physical anorexic body only [...] the exclusion of the anorexic mind from bio-medicine's professional jurisdiction can be seen as reflecting the existing in-built structure within the medical profession […] The challenge was how to produce standardized and formalized knowledge, the hallmark of scientific medicine. (2002:467–72)

This search for standardised and formalised knowledge has continued until the present and is reflected in the development of 'scientifically' validated psychiatric rating instruments, such as the Eating Disorders Inventory (Garner et al, 1983b). The EDI is used chiefly as a research and screening tool, as an aid to, rather than a substitute for, the doctor's clinical judgement. It is based on diagnostic criteria enshrined in the 'bible' of psychiatric disorders, the *Diagnostic and Statistical Manual* (DSM), (APA, 1994). The DSM comprises 'certain' criteria, which must be present for a diagnosis to be made. In the case of anorexia, the diagnosis is defined as follows:

> A. Refusal to maintain body weight at or above a minimally normal weight for age and height (e.g. weight loss leading to maintenance of body weight less than 85% of that expected, or failure to make expected weight gain during period of growth leading to body weight less than 85% of that expected);
>
> B. Intense fear of gaining weight or becoming fat, even though underweight;
>
> C. Disturbance in the way in which one's body weight or shape is experienced, undue influence of body weight or shape on self-evaluation, or denial of the seriousness of the current low body weight;
>
> D. In postmenarcheal females, amenorrhea, i.e. the absence of at least three consecutive menstrual cycles (a woman is considered to have amenorrhea if her periods only follow hormone, e.g. estrogen, administration).

From the above criteria, we can observe that psychiatrists emphasise 'fear of weight gain' as the *sine qua non* for anorexia to be diagnosed. The diagnostic rules applied to anorexia centre almost entirely on 'fat phobia'. Two of the criteria described above (A and D) relate solely to physiological processes (generally loss of weight, but also cessation of the menses), while only criteria B and C focus on psychological concerns. Even these psychological criteria however, describe unelaborated cognitive states, where the sufferer experiences intense fear of gaining weight or becoming fat as well as 'disturbance in the way [...] one's body weight [...] is experienced'. Where this fear or disturbance may have arisen from remains unexplored.

Diagnostic criteria are important in medicine, since without them a correct diagnosis could not be made. A degree of 'abstraction' is thus inevitable in the diagnostic process. Also it often desirable to establish diagnostic certainty. If incorrectly diagnosed, patients may experience significant problems, (such as incarceration). For these reasons, the positivist approach has become privileged in psychiatry and doctors internalise this approach as part of their socialisation into the world of medicine. Such an approach however may influence the doctor's responses to the patient in the illness consultation. Doctors may thus be persuaded to concentrate on the technical, at the expense of the personal or social aspects of the patient's condition.

The technical criteria in the psychiatric 'bible'– the DSM – therefore constitute 'ultimate truths' (Kutchins and Kirk, 1997). As Rowe explains:

> The DSM discusses neither cause nor cure. The whole of the DSM reflects the desire to pin down and to categorize the flux of human experience rather than to enter into it in the hope of understanding how another person perceives himself [sic] and his world. In psychiatry twas ever thus. In that other bible of the profession, *Clinical Psychiatry*, the authors Elliot Slater and Martin Roth, great names in the pantheon of British psychiatry, advised their fellow psychiatrists that, 'It is the objective world in which we live and to which the subjective world must pay deference. It is more important to know what the facts are than what the patient makes of them' [Slater and Roth, 1969]. This is actually a claim to possess a superhuman power to know the Absolute Truth, to perceive reality directly, unimpeded by the interpretations which mere human beings have to make of a reality which is forever beyond their grasp. (1997:xvi–xvii)

This claim to superhuman power may lead psychiatry into prioritising its own definitions of the patient's problem over the sufferer's common sense experience (Bury, 1988, Kleinman, 1988, Mishler, 1984, Strauss et al, 1984). Many doctors, however, apply diagnostic criteria subtly to accommodate variation in individual cases. But even this concern for individuality takes place within the context of an over-arching template, which tends to emphasise 'certainty' and 'objectivity' and which minimises the search for alternative (possibly social) explanations.

Technical criteria in the DSM emphasise 'fat phobia'. 'Fat phobia' encapsulates the emphasis which psychiatrists place on bodily concerns in diagnosing anorexia. A further logical question is whether other symptoms in the psychiatric canon are also privileged in diagnosing the illness, and whether these symptoms are any more helpful and accurate than 'fear of weight gain' in uncovering the full range of potential explanations for the disorder. While DSM criteria centre almost entirely on weight, in other psychiatric fora (Lawrence, 1995, Bruch, 1973), a further symptom has been identified as key to the causes and presentation of anorexia. This symptom is 'fear of maturity', wherein anorexia is described as flight from the responsibilities and independence of adulthood. The anorexic's mother, this symptom argues, has failed to instill a strong sense of self in her daughter, and has thus failed to prepare her for the demands of adult life. Fear of fatness and fear of maturity therefore, constitute two elements of a stereotype applied by clinicians to the assessment of anorexia. A full description of this stereotype will now be presented.

The Anorexic Stereotype

The cognitive stereotype

'Fear of maturity' forms a pivotal element of the 'anorexic stereotype'. It features centrally in established anorexia rating instruments such as the Eating Disorders Inventory (EDI) (Garner et al, 1983b), and together with 'fear of weight gain', forms a central premise of the clinical model of anorexia . It is interesting to examine why symptoms such as 'fear of maturity' and 'fear of fatness' remain so privileged in psychiatry. I argue that this is because such criteria are the product of a socially negotiated process (engaged in by psychiatrists), rather than concrete manifestations in the objective world. In socially negotiating the diagnosis of anorexia, psychiatrists have 'constructed' the typical cognitive profile of the anorexic. This book seeks to examine whether this profile is supported by data.

The demographic stereotype

As well as stereotyping the anorexic's cognitive state, clinicians have also tended to stereotype the demographic profile of the anorexic. She is frequently presented as a middle class youngster, (Morgan and Russell, 1975), with good educational qualifications (Hamburg and Herzog, 1985), and it is sometimes suggested that she will live in a big city (Nadoka et al, 1996). A key element of the anorexic stereotype concerns the age of the typical sufferer. Anorexics are usually reported to be very young women (Halmi et al 1979). In addition, they are almost exclusively depicted as female (Robinson and Holden, 1986). Since the earliest commentaries on the disorder were published (Bruch, 1978), this stereotype of the anorexic has persisted. (Lucas et al, 1988, Hoek and Brook, 1985, Azuma and Henmi, 1982, Crisp et al, 1976, Morgan and Russell, 1975). In addition, anorexics have been described as obedient adolescents who excel academically (Hoek and Brook, 1985, Eagles et al, 1990). Anorexics are thus presented as educationally successful, consistent with the model of the sufferer as a studious, dutiful, but educationally pressurised young woman.

The Social Nature of Psychiatric Criteria

Like all knowledge, the criteria used to define anorexia are inseparable from the society in which they develop. As society changes so also do the criteria. Such an analysis integrates the individual's experience of ill health with the wider society from which that individual comes. Psychiatry conversely, tends to remove suffering from the social context in which it occurs. In so doing it pursues a 'reductionist biological discourse uncritically' (Lee, 1996:22). This 'reductionist discourse' leads psychiatry to search for closed ended 'certain' criteria. These criteria, however, are modified over time, to reflect the prevailing values of successive social moments.

Psychiatrists, however, tend to be reluctant to engage with an appraisal of this social construction of disease categories (Hepworth, 1999) and have largely failed to examine the process by which specific diagnostic criteria are socially negotiated. This should not altogether surprise us. Such a situation may be observed in any discipline. Sociology for example, as well as medicine, also has its own knowledge base, which it defends vigorously. The sociological perspective privileges social explanations, for example, while declaring 'natural' explanations invalid (Elston, 1997). Sociologists are thus apt to criticise scientific 'essentialism' in others, while adopting social essentialism in their own work (Woolgar, 1988). The sociologist's critique of science is therefore just as socially situated as the scientific knowledge it criticises.

It is important to acknowledge that my own perspective is itself informed by this very sociological essentialism and it is important that the reader is aware of this. The critiquing of my own epistemology while simultaneously applying such epistemology, however, is a bit like trying to 'push a bus which one is riding' (Berger and Luckmann,

1966:25). Nevertheless if one is to be reflexive in one's own approach it is important to show awareness of one's own inconsistencies and contradictions. While pointing out the pitfalls of scientific essentialism we must remain reflexive about our own position, and allow the reader to evaluate our findings in light of this. If we are honest and reflexive about our own essentialism, our critique of other forms of essentialism will be all the more valid.

Towards a Feminist and Sociological Analysis of Anorexia

Building on existing sociological work (Locker, 2003, 1983, MacSween, 1993, Bury, 1988, Kleinman, 1988, Mishler, 1984, Strauss et al, 1984), this book offers a sociological and feminist analysis of anorexia nervosa. Both perspectives have themselves emerged as forms of knowledge over the past 150 years, and one should be wary of implying that such approaches are especially qualified to judge the merits of psychiatry. Nevertheless these are the perspectives I have selected as they reflect my own theoretical orientation as well as 'uncovering' the development of 'anorexic knowledge'. The feminist approach uncovers the male-defined nature of such knowledge (Harding, 1991, Fox-Keller, 1985), while the sociological approach identifies how diagnoses are socially produced (Helman, 2000, Kleinman, 1988, Bury, 1988). Such approaches thus accommodate an appraisal of the causes as well as the presentation of the disorder. In this way the book will avoid the 'easy answers' put forward in the DSM model of the fat phobic anorexic.

The DSM is a basic template to which doctors are taught to adhere when making a diagnosis. Its criteria, as clinicians readily acknowledge, represent a basic minimum, which the patient must exhibit to be diagnosed with the disorder. As such, DSM criteria may be considered as the basic symptoms of anorexia nervosa. On top of this, doctors are also taught to consider broad underlying causes, emphasising personality, family background, fear of maturity, self-esteem, class and educational level (Bruch, 1978, Crisp, 1995, Crisp et al, 1976). Doctors themselves are therefore well aware of the distinction between basic minimum symptoms and the broader underlying causes of anorexia. Nevertheless, clinical descriptions of causes as well as symptoms tend to be presented with a high degree of certainty (see Crisp, 1995, for example).

In a book such as this, it is important to examine the distinction between symptoms and causes. It may be argued that in anorexia there is an extensive overlap between the two. For example, if we take the key symptom of control – i.e. the contention that anorexia manifests as a profound desire to exercise control over eating, we notice that this symptom is also a cause of the illness – the sufferer becomes ill because she wishes to control food (the symptom) to offset a lack of control in other areas of her life (the cause). In this book there may thus be some overlap in my discussion of symptoms and causes. This is inevitable, given the organic link between symptoms and causes in an illness such as anorexia.

If anorexia is about loss of control, then the complex social context in which loss of control occurs needs to be analysed. This may be achieved by adopting a feminist approach. The social debasement which women experience – through e.g. discrimination at work, domestic violence, and sexual exploitation – and the loss of control attendant on such experiences are incorporated in a feminist analysis of anorexia. Feminism thus facilitates an analysis of anorexia that includes an appraisal of women's disempowerment. It emphasises the social experiences of unequal pay, inequality in the family, and the unequal and objectified representation of women's bodies in the media. By deploying such an analysis we can appraise not only the psychological presentation of anorexia, but also the social causes which contribute to the development of the illness.

It is important to acknowledge that it is not only physicians who have developed a stereotype of the anorexic. A feminist approach is used in this book, but such an approach is not faultless. Feminists themselves have produced an archetype which constructs the sufferer as a political protester reacting against society's oppression of women (Orbach, 1993, MacSween, 1993, Hepworth, 1999). The feminist stereotype however, is arguably less powerful than the clinical model and its impact has been largely restricted to academic circles. The medical stereotype, conversely, has pervaded public consciousness and the media, as well as the clinical setting. For this reason, the priority of sociology must be to deconstruct and theorise the clinical stereotype.

It is also important to mention one area that this book does not propose to discuss. It does not propose to analyse patient testimony from a psychoanalytical perspective. The project identifies the manner in which anorexia is constructed as a social entity. As a result, the book avoids appraising patient testimonies from a purely psychological point of view, focusing instead on aspects of these testimonies which are of sociological interest. The book does not therefore contain psychoanalytical evaluations, and makes no reference to neo-psychoanalytical perspectives, such as psychoanalytical feminism.

The Story of the Anorexic Stereotype: A Summary

To summarise the issues described so far, the chapter has argued that over the centuries, medicine has constructed an archetype of anorexia, influenced by the predominance of specific psychiatric approaches at a given time. In the nineteenth century, with the growth of scientific medicine, the case study approach allowed anorexia to be identified as an illness. Subsequent developments in psychiatric knowledge changed the manner in which anorexia was understood, culminating in the standardised (though simultaneously multi-disciplinary) approaches in place today. Currently, anorexia is viewed in stereotypical terms. The anorexic stereotype concerns the symptoms associated with anorexia and the type of person who develops it. With regards to the symptoms associated with the disorder, medicine privileges fear of fatness and fear of maturity. In relation to the type of person who develops the disease, medicine suggests that the anorexic is typically a young, middle-class, high achiever, possibly from a big city.

The current chapter has discussed the social production of 'anorexic knowledge'. The production of anorexic knowledge has resulted in the creation of labels (such as 'fat phobic') which are applied to the anorexic patient. In the next chapter, the labeling of anorexic patients is discussed with reference to research from the field of chronic illness. Chapter 2 therefore analyses the experience of anorexia as a long-term disorder. The chapter begins however, with a discussion of what we currently know about food, eating, diet, the body and anorexia. It is to a discussion of these issues that I now turn.

Chapter 2
A Review of Sociological Literature in Food, Eating and Anorexia

Introduction

In this chapter sociological literature in the area of food, eating, and anorexia, is discussed. Given the central symbolic significance of food (and food avoidance) to the anorexic, the chapter focuses initially on the sociology of food. It then explores the subject of eating, particularly in relation to the differences in eating behaviour between men and women. Dieting is subsequently discussed and (since people diet to alter the shape of their bodies), a brief discussion of the sociology of the body follows.

The second half of the chapter focuses entirely on the subject of anorexia. Anorexia is discussed with reference to current feminist and sociological theory. More specifically however, it is discussed in the context of the sociology of chronic illness. Anorexia is a long-term disorder and insights from research into chronic illness can usefully be applied to its study. Such research suggests that certain diagnoses may symbolise certain things to the sufferer. Anorexia may symbolise that sufferers have a serious psychiatric disorder. Also of key symbolic value to the anorexic is the issue of food.

Food

Research into the sociology of food has markedly increased in recent years (Warde, 1997, Mennell, !996, Germov and Williams, 2004, Lupton, 1996a) suggesting that the study of food in sociology has 'come of age'. It is appropriate to ask why the discipline has only recently become a focus of research in sociology. Mennell (2004) argues that the ascendancy of the discipline can be explained as a result of the gains of feminism:

> For most of the twentieth century the prestigious topics tended to be stratification and class inequality, politics and power, industrial organization and bureaucracy. All were in some sense masculine concerns. The inequality between the sexes was taken for granted, while that between social strata was not: work was mainly a man's world, the home and the kitchen a woman's. (2004:vi)

As women's concerns began to be accorded equal status, the study of food became established in sociology (Mennell, 2004). Food, however was always a focus of interest to anthropologists (Douglas, 1972). This interest may have reflected a paternalistic assumption that 'primitive' societies rest on 'simple' structures such as food exchange, while the social organisation of 'advanced' societies was more complex. But the key reason for the rise in the study of food nevertheless appears to be the 'profound effect' which feminism 'undoubtedly had on the sociological enterprise as a whole' (Mennell, 2004:vi). Such a development, however, does not tell the whole story. The success of the sociology of food was also the result of a shift in sociological focus from the 'primacy of production to the primacy of consumption' (Mennell, 2004:vi). Issues such as taste and lifestyle in the area of food, (and in other areas), now became a focus in sociology (Bourdieu, 1994). Giddens (1991), for example, explains that people use the lifestyle they adopt to establish a self-identity which they communicate to others. Taste in food is a key element of this identity.

Food is also of intense symbolic significance to the anorexic who structures her life around its avoidance. It is thus important in this book to assess food's symbolic nature and an exposition of this issue will now be offered.

The Symbolic Position of Food

Atkinson emphasises food's symbolic function. 'There are [...] a number of symbolic or semantic spaces that seem particularly well demarcated by the concrete representation of food stuffs' (1983:11). Atkinson discusses symbolism with particular reference to the wholesome and natural image of healthfoods, but it is in Twigg's (1983) discussion of meat and vegetarianism that food symbolism is most closely examined. At the time Twigg was writing, meat was the most highly prized of food, the centre around which a meal is based, a metonym for food itself. The most valued meat was red meat whose power was derived from associations with strength, muscle, aggression, passion and sexuality. Red meat enjoyed this symbolism partly because of its association with blood – which is itself of intense symbolic significance, denoting inheritance and signifying personal characteristics such as hot or noble blood.

The symbolism of blood and its association with meat exemplifies food's semiotic significance. Such symbolism allows food to act as an integrating mechanism. Drinks, for example may be shared with workmen, but meals are given only to family and friends. Social occasions, as Douglas, (1972), explains, are encoded by the type of food consumed. Meals are ordered in a scale of importance, from Christmas and Sunday dinners at the highest end of the hierarchy to tea and biscuits at the bottom (Charles and Kerr, 1988). This formal ordering of meals reflects the increased social patterning and control required in eating. Elias (1978) thus described the social evolution of certain forms of table manners which constructed certain activities as normal (e.g. eating with a knife and fork) and other, hitherto widely practiced, activities (e.g. eating with the hands, or 'throwing food', etc.) as unacceptable.

Table manners and the scheduling of specific meals (e.g. Sunday dinner) at specific times are all mechanisms through which an 'ideal' of family life is structured. This ideal, described as 'family ideology' by Charles and Kerr (1988:17) is underpinned by the social roles each family member occupies. The provision of food, clearly identified as the woman's task, can viewed as a symbol of relations of power and subordination existing in the family.

A key aspect of a woman's obligation to her family is to provide a 'proper meal' for her husband and children (Charles and Kerr, 1988:17). The 'proper meal' usually of meat, potatoes and vegetables (or other food in different ethnic groups, (Bush et al, 1998)), is 'constitutive of the family as a cohesive social unit' (Charles and Kerr, 1988:21). Where a mother fails to provide 'proper meals' she is not a proper mother and her family is not a proper family. Perhaps unsurprisingly, women feel pressurised into preparing 'proper meals' (Charles and Kerr, 1988).

Nowadays its is often suggested that the 'proper' meal is in decline, and has been replaced by an 'empire of snacks' (Fischler, 1980:946). 'Microwave ovens, TV dinners, etc. makes it relatively easy for anyone, regardless of culinary skill, to get a meal, or a substitute for a meal, at irregular times', (Warde, 1997:71). While this trend has certainly increased in recent decades (Fischler, 1980:946), it is important to emphasise that proper meals are still provided on a regular basis (Warde,1997). TV dinners are inferior in flavour to freshly cooked food and nutrition experts criticise 'convenience' eating (Royal College of Physicians, 2004, Health Education Council, 1983). Also, restaurant meals are viewed as weekly treats that provide no more than a temporary respite from the routine of cooking (Warde, 1997). Quick, convenient meals have yet to replace the proper meal and it is appropriate to ask why.

The majority of women studied by Charles and Kerr (1988) and Warde (1997) continued to prepare proper meals regardless of the cost to themselves in terms of time. These women were very aware of the expressive nature of food provision. In preparing food for their families these women were saying, 'I love you'. Warde (1997) suggests that the linking of food with the expression of love, while being something women may take pride in, nevertheless increases the subordination of women in the home and in society. By constructing women's role as one of servicing the family (with those falling short in this task presumably not loving their husbands and children), women's subordination is thus reinforced.

> Means exist for reducing time spent on domestic food production [...] A diet exclusively comprised of packaged and prepared foods from the supermarket [...] would save time and effort. At a price all meals could be purchased ready-made in restaurants: the early feminist vision of the kitchenless home is now a viable commercial alternative. However it is unlikely that such alternatives [...] would be generally acceptable [...] there is something suspicious or improper about convenience food. (Warde, 1997:131–52)

Women's magazines (Warde, 1997) therefore suggest that 'convenience' can be attained by 'spreading the load' (preparing food at a more leisurely time and freezing) not because women lack the skill but because they have other even more pressing things to do. In Warde's study of magazines, storage tips were emphasised in the recipe columns, but the expectation was always that women would cook fresh food, if not from scratch, then from food they had prepared earlier 'thus suggesting that care and convenience might be reconciled', (1997:136).

Women therefore balance the provision of care (in the form of freshly cooked food) with the time demands of other equally pressing activities (such as earning money for the family). The cooking suggestions made in recipe columns (e.g. partial cooking and freezing when time permits) indicate that women try assiduously to provide as much care as possible in the time available.

> Although almost all household foods are now bought, the transformation of groceries into meals often requires considerable time, effort and skill [...] despite the enormous application of technology to the home, the amount of domestic work that women have to do seems not to decrease. (Warde, 1997:126)

Home cooked lunches and breakfasts may have declined, but the proper meal, prepared in the evening, (Warde, 1997) continues to form a key mechanism around which the routines of family life are structured.

Nevertheless, it is undeniable that 'convenience' foods are widely used (Fischler, 1980). Mennell however, suggests that this may have done little to save women time. Rather the effect has been to put a more varied range of food items within the reach of the 'ordinary housewife', thus markedly improving the nation's diet. Such foods so often seen as undermining cookery skills and traditions, have also played a vital part in committing 'housewives to be more adventurous and varied in their cooking', (1996:261).

Ritzer, (1996) also notes the increased choice offered by convenience food. 'People', Ritzer explains, 'can readily extract a wide range of ingredients [from the freezer] when needed' (1996:52). But few would deny that even where 'efficient' pre-packaged pastry or frozen peas are used, the process of putting a meal on the table for a family of four after a hard day's work is an onerous task, and one almost always performed by women (Charles and Kerr, 1988).

Food – The Division of Labour in the Household

Sociological studies have therefore found that domestic work, including food provision, is overwhelmingly performed by women (Warde, 1997, Oakley, 1976). Some sociologists (Warde and Heatherington, 1994) argue that today men do more housework than their fathers, but nevertheless women continue to do significantly more than men. Because women perform most food preparation, the social patterning accompanying the provision of food has particular relevance for the social organisation of women's lives. DeVault (1991) suggests that such work produces the 'life of the group', while simultaneously confining women to a subordinate role. Warde however suggests that this arrangement now makes men feel guilty.

> A hard pressed housewife [however] might get little comfort from the fact that her husband now feels guilty about his limited contribution. Nevertheless it

> confirms that the stereotypical response of an earlier generation of men [...] is now very much a minority opinion. (1997:144)

Food as a Site of Conflict

The role of providing 'proper meals' therefore falls to women. A refusal to eat such food, on the part of the anorexic daughter, is a powerful form of protest – a disintegrating strategy that strikes at the heart of family life. Food may therefore be used as a way of expressing conflict. The focus on food as a site of conflict was analysed by Ellis (1983). Ellis illustrates the importance of food as symbolic of the relationships within violent families. For violent men 'the women's role in meal provision is a symbolic as well as material task' (Ellis, 1983:164). In other words, meal provision is part of the contract to which the battered wife acceded when she agreed to marry. Burgoyne and Clark's (1983) discussion of step-families also describes how food is used as a site of conflict. Step-children are reported as criticising the food provided by their step-parent as a method of focusing personal dislike.

Just as food is symbolic of family life (and its breakdown), the regular provision of meals is seen as an occasion where all members of the family can be together. Food provides not only a link between family members, but is also indicative of the link between the natural and the social. Indeed so fundamental is the link between food and the social world that food is often used as a metaphor for society. Health foods, for example, with their emphasis on wholesome values and an outdoor lifestyle, may be seen to symbolise an alternative method of social organisation (Atkinson, 1983), based on clean living, regular habits, and a moral approach to society.

Food – the Boundary between Nature and Culture

Food mediates between nature and culture. It can be seen as a metaphor for the 'many different ways in which the worlds of culture – of meanings, values and human work – are created and sustained in the face of an alien, non-human universe' (Atkinson, 1983:11). Quoting Levi Strauss, Atkinson explains, 'we cook to demonstrate that we are civilised men [sic] and not animals' (Atkinson, 1983:11). Similarly, Twigg (1983) explains that cooking is an essential variable in the meat based food hierarchy. 'Tearing at raw flesh with one's teeth is an image of horror suitable to monsters and the semi human' (1983:25).

Cooking therefore, is a cultural process, transforming raw material from nature into culture (Lupton, 1996a). When we consume food, Lupton explains, we consume the cultural universe (1996a:16). Cooked food is a linking substance between the two worlds of nature and society, 'the human and the natural, the outside and the inside' (Lupton, 1996a:17). Sharing a meal is therefore a central integrating mechanism in both 'primitive' and modern societies. The social structure is unified and lubricated through partaking of food, and the cultural importance of eating is highly significant.

Food as a Moral Issue

The emphasis on right and wrong choices in relation to food highlights the underlying moral dimension associated with food and eating. Atkinson suggests that health foods convey 'the message that social order and personal virtue can be eaten [...] their purchase is thus portrayed as a morally desirable act' (Atkinson, 1983:16). Atkinson also explains that specific food practices have moral underpinnings. Vegetarian philosophy, for example, focuses on both animal welfare and on the welfare of the environment. This is particularly relevant in relation to the expense of meat production, where the immorality of animal exploitation is related to the immorality of exploiting the third world (Atkinson, 1983).

This propensity for investing food with moral significance was also evident in Blaxter and Paterson's (1983) discussion of food meanings across two generations in Scotland. Good foods, in the view of the older generation, were 'prepared in basic ways by boiling or baking, and never tinned or highly processed' (1983:96). Such careful preparation of food would suggest that an equal amount of care and ceremony might be applied when the food is eaten. Considerations governing how people eat are central to a text on anorexia and sociological research in this area will now be described.

Eating

In any text which discusses anorexia, it is appropriate to examine sociological research in the area of eating. Elias (1978) explains that, as society became more affluent and complex, table manners became more formal and refined. The gorging, belching and spitting of the medieval banquet was thus replaced by socially patterned behaviour, reflecting a more complex society. In the medieval period, the normal experience was one of subsistence and famine. By the seventeenth and eighteenth centuries food supplies were secured as a result of state formation, pacification and trade, allowing even poor people to occasionally eat well:

> Once food supplies were more plentiful and reliable the aristocratic 'blow out' stopped. This means of asserting distance between themselves and the upstarts immediately beneath them in the social hierarchy reached its physical limit. Groaning boards became vulgar, ever more elaborate concoctions the height of good taste. More internalized self control became valued. This was eventually reflected in the social disapproval of obesity [...] and, for females especially, the social pressure towards self-restraint and ever thinner body images has been associated with a rising incidence of eating disorders. (Mennell et al, 1994:17)

With the growing security of food supplies, a discerning palate, (rather than a voracious appetite) became the mark of nobility. The most modern expression of this development is nouvelle cuisine. Such cuisine, with its 'huge cost, minimal food and emphasis on decoration is [therefore] conspicuous waste' (Warde, 1997:104).

It is not only in the area of etiquette that specific groups apply rules to eating. With regard to the amount of food consumed men and women behave differently. Williams and Germov (2004) explain that because society values thinness, women's eating patterns are often governed by the desire to remain thin. Women and men thus eat in a different way. Researchers have identified specific gender patterns in eating (Williams and Germov, 2004) and have described the contradictory orientation which women have towards food, (Williams and Germov, 2004). These contradictions relate particularly to women's perception of their bodies, but also to their role as food providers (Lawrence, 1995). As indicated in the previous section, women often consider meal provision to be their responsibility and may prioritise the nutritional needs of others over their own. As a result, to care for others and to maintain a slender body, women may be permanently conscious of a need to suppress their own appetites.

Mennell explains that appetite and hunger may be regarded as two separate entities. Hunger is biological. It is a bodily function which alerts humans to the need to 're-fuel' by consuming food. Appetite however may be viewed as psychological and social. 'We tend to think of hunger, appetite and eating as directly linked in a simple chain of causality [but this] omits the internal processes though which a person constitutes his [sic] act', (Mennell, 1996:21). These internal processes (e.g. fear of weight gain) may influence the manner in which a person eats. The social constitution of appetite may therefore cause eating to be set at a particular level to ensure a socially desirable body. Mennell calls this socially constructed appetite an 'appestat'. For women, 'appestats' are likely to be set at low. Historically however, appestats may have been set at high, as larger figures were acceptable and the consumption of huge amounts (as a respite from famine) was encouraged.

When food and money are scarce, this will undoubtedly affect the amount and type of food eaten. Conversely, for more affluent groups a wider variety of food is available. Nouvelle cuisine provides an example by which differences in eating may be used by certain classes to distinguish themselves from those they consider inferior, and an appraisal of class and eating will now be offered.

Class and eating

Several sociologists have examined the issue of class differences in eating (Mennell, 1996, Bourdieu, 1994, Warde, 1997). Warde acknowledges the existence of social differences suggesting that

> a good deal of social difference [...] can be appreciated simply in terms of income and expenditure [...] richer households spend much more money in absolute terms than do poorer households, while that constitutes a significantly smaller proportion of their total expenditure. (1997:124)

Class distinction in the area of food was described by Bourdieu (1984, 1994). Bourdieu identified the extent to which tastes in food are divided along class lines. The middle class are not only richer but also claim that they are culturally superior, (and therein lies their power). Among the working class, Bourdieu observed the 'taste of necessity [...] produced by conditions of existence that rule out all alternatives [...] and leave no choice but the taste for the necessary' (1994:178). In Bourdieu's view working class people have no choice and hence no taste. Were they to be given the choice, however, their taste would quickly develop.

The link between social class (particularly income) and food provision has also been emphasised by Charles and Kerr (1988). Women in higher social classes are much more likely to prioritise the goodness of food, while those from lower socio economic groups are understandably concerned with cost. The differences between 'working' and 'middle' class eating has frequently been noted by sociologists (Warde, 1997, Graham, 1984). Warde (1997), for example, suggests even though food is now more varied, class differences in food persist. However Mennell (1996) argues that these differences are diminishing, with middle class tastes permeating all social groups.

It is hard however, to fundamentally change eating behaviour (Warde, 1997). While families often eat 'exotic' food for a change, 'traditional' foods nevertheless make up most of their diet (Ilmonen, 1991, Warde, 1997). Indeed television cooks such as Gary Rhodes (2001) and Anthony Worrall-Thompson (2003) emphasise the wholesomeness and palatability of 'traditional' British food, which they encode as symbolic of an earlier and better social order. What is perceived as traditional may be created by the media, and dishes so designated have become very heterogeneous (Warde, 1997). 'Behind invented tradition', Warde explains, 'lurks the imagined community a site of social group membership that promise collective security and group identity', (1997:66). In most of Warde's Manchester sample women preferred to serve 'traditional' food as a 'comforting antidote to [...] innovation' (1997:66). With so much choice nowadays, individuals may not be confident about what to select (Fischler,1980) and may wish to find some certainties to 'cling to'. This certainty may be found in traditional food.

In summary, Warde supports Bourdieu's suggestion of distinction between middle and working class, while Mennell believes that contrasts between classes and the way they eat are 'diminishing' with an increasing variety of food now available to everyone. In view of this, it might be supposed that the food habits of the middle and working class are beginning to converge in the area of food consumption. In the area of food restriction also, it is possible that working class and middle class behaviour is converging, with thin bodies increasingly being viewed by all classes as desirable (Gard and Freeman, 1996). While dieting behaviour between classes may be converging however, attitudes to dieting between men and women are sharply differentiated. In relation to gender, dieting behaviour is clearly organised on sex specific lines (Williams and Germov, 2004) and a discussion of dieting, particularly in relation to women, is now presented.

Dieting

As indicated earlier, to achieve a socially acceptable body shape, women eat in a different way to men. As Williams and Germov explain, 'gendered eating behaviour is epitomised by the sexual division of dieting. Dieting is primarily a female act' (2004:340). For this reason (and also because this is a book about anorexia) it is appropriate to discuss dieting at this point in the text. Researchers have suggested that dieting may be a permanent occupation for many women (Lawrence, 1995, Orbach, 1993, Bordo, 1993, Williams and Germov, 2004) resulting in 'a lifelong "tug of war" with food' (Williams and Germov, 2004:339). Women's eating is therefore mediated by social images of the desirable body and consequently many women's relationship to food is characterised by guilt, self-denial and despair. Studies have indicated that many women are unhappy with their weight (Lawrence, 1995, Orbach, 1993) and the number of young women currently on a diet has been estimated to be as high as 50% (Williams and Gerrmov, 2004). As Williams and Germov explain however, more women than men are within their healthy weight range, and women therefore have fewer health reasons for dieting than men.

It is therefore appropriate to ask why women continue to diet. As Orbach (1993) and Bordo (1993) indicate, the slimming, fashion and beauty industries create an unrealistic ideal to which women are taught to aspire. Such an ideal may be impossible to attain, and consequently the demand for dieting and beauty products which promise success is infinite. Some researchers however (Bordo, 1993) suggest that women may pursue this ideal for positive reasons (see page 49). For these women, the attainment of the ideal body may be a source of pleasure and empowerment. Nevertheless, dieting remains a predominantly female activity in which food denial and weight monitoring may become a way of life. As Williams and Germov explain 'A sexual division of dieting exists' (2004:360) in which those on a diet are usually women.

Dieting may become so central to women that it may begin to resemble a military campaign. As Warde explains:

> People adopt dietary programmes from books and magazines. They [join clubs] count calories [...] display charts [...] weigh themselves on bathroom scales regularly. They use tape measures or waistbands [...] to detect alterations in size. They enter upon crash diets [and] the vocabulary of war is never far distant. (Warde, 1997:94)

Warde is correct in his assertion that 'the vocabulary of war is never far distant'. A recent 'slimfast' advertising campaign from 2004 featured four bikini clad models striking a determined pose, with a legend reading 'we will fight them on the beaches', (in reference to slimmer women with whom the models needed to compete). Similarly, in the 1980s, the low calorie crispbread company 'Ryvita' coined the term 'the inchwar'. This battleground mentality is part of an ongoing campaign to mould the body into a superthin identity.

Concern with slimming and weight control is now commonplace in women's magazines (Warde, 1997), where low fat recipes are now listed as a matter of course. While the sale of healthy foodstuffs has increased (Warde, 1997), so also has the sale of unhealthy, indulgent treats such as chocolate. Such an 'antimony' between self-denial and hedonism is logical. 'As you master the flesh, you also need respite from the asceticism', (Warde, 1997:92). Such respite increases 'guilt, concern, [and] self measurement', (1997:92), thus setting the process of self-denial, indulgence and self-denial in train once more. Women worry about how much food they eat because of how this will make their bodies look. Since food intake is regulated by women in order to mould their bodies, it is now appropriate to briefly discuss the sociology of the body.

As Germov and Williams explain, 'regimes of bodily control, particularly in the regulation of food intake are now common features of Western culture' (2004:336). Germov and Williams refer to such regimes as 'healthism, an ideology that views health as the primary human goal' (2004:336). Much research has shown that chubby, fat and especially obese bodies are socially viewed in highly negative terms (Fabricatore and Wadden, 2004, Annis et al, 2003, Brownwell and Fairburn, 1995). Such bodies are equated with lack of control, sloth, loneliness and even immorality (Fabricatore and Walden, 2004). In Western society the ideal body is thin. This ideal, initially reflected in the boyish figure of the 1920s flapper (Lawrence, 1995) was later superseded by a more voluptuous stereotype exemplified by Marilyn Monroe (Lawrence, 1995). In the 1960s however the thin ideal (reflected in the figures of models like Twiggy) became fully established and the ideal body has since become thinner and thinner (Lawrence, 1995, Garner et al, 1980).

In patriarchal society, the shape of women's bodies is therefore a public matter. A patriarchal imperative exhorts women to achieve a thin body. Such an ideal represents an attempt to control the bodies of women. In earlier centuries, such control was physical (Williams and Germov, 2004). Women wore constructive garments, such as corsets and long skirts, and their bodies were prohibited from entering certain social spaces. Nowadays the control is internal. It is 'exercised [...] through the internalisation of the thin ideal' (Williams and Germov, 2004:346). Some sociologists though, have stressed that women are not simply 'passive dopes' responding to patriarchal pressures (Bordo, 1993). In striving for a thin, toned body, women are using their own agency to achieve an image which is a source of pleasure and pride. 'It is women themselves who practice this discipline on and against their own bodies [...] This self-surveillance is a form of obedience to patriarchy' (Wearing, 1996:88, cited in Williams and Germov, 2004: 341), but one where women discern advantages in their willingness to conform. 'Discipline [therefore] becomes individualized and internalized' (Warde, 1997:93). Of course there is external pressure to be slim but nevertheless 'this remains more a matter of self discipline than state intervention', (Warde, 1997:93).

> Dieting and the pursuit of the thin ideal can thus be viewed as a rational response by women striving for acceptance in the context of the dominant ideals of beauty, sexuality and femininity. The internalization of patriarchal norms explain the active role women play in perpetuating the thin ideal [...] Women police their own bodies and the bodies of other women in a system of surveillance [...] this process of women's body monitoring [may be described] as the 'body panopticon' effect. (Williams and Germov, 2004:355–6)

Sociologists who stress the importance 'body panopticism' and 'self-surveillance' are largely from the post structuralist school (Foucault, 1979, Bordo, 1993). Post-structuralists are especially concerned with the effects of power on the body. For this reason 'embodiment' is central to the post-structuralist position. Foucault, arguably the founder of post-structuralism, has placed the body at the centre of his work. The body, Foucault tells us, is 'directly involved in a political field; power relations have an immediate hold upon it; they invest it, mark it, train it, torture it, force it to carry out tasks, to perform ceremonies, to emit signs' (Foucault,1979:25). These relations of power permeate through to the micro-elements of society. The formation of this power is dynamic. It is dispersed through network of relations permanently in flux. This 'mechanics of power' defines:

> how one may have a hold over others' bodies, not only so that they may do what one wishes, but so that they may operate as one wishes, with the techniques, the speed and the efficiency that one determines. (Foucault, 1979:138)

The body, Foucault explains, is historically constituted. Under capitalism, it has become the focus of numerous powerful agencies, namely medicine, the social survey and the beauty and fitness industry. This has given rise to the system of surveillance, referred to as panopticism (see above). Like Foucault, Lupton (1994) also views the body as a social construction, affected by 'discursive processes and power struggles' (1994:20). The human body, Lupton explains, has a history – it has been represented differently at different times and is treated differently and lived differently. Such issues have become important in sociology, where the sociology of the body is currently very much in vogue. Embodiment, however, is of only peripheral relevance to the current text. This may appear paradoxical, as, at first glance, anorexia is a bodily disorder. However, I am concerned with knowledge in relation to psychological, rather than bodily, constructs. These constructs include obsessionalism and control, symptoms which are not centrally located in the body. Though I also discuss weight phobia (a bodily symptom), I argue that psychiatry places a disproportionate emphasis on this symptom. For this reason I have minimised my own focus on the sociology of the body, preferring to concentrate instead on the discursive construction of knowledge surrounding anorexia. Since the concept of anorexia is so central to the research described in this text, a discussion of sociological understanding in the area of anorexia will now be offered.

Anorexia

This is a book on the subject of anorexia and therefore it is important to discuss anorexia as part of this literature review. Anorexia is usually estimated to affect about 1% of women (Hepworth, 2004), and 0.05% of men, (Robinson and Holden, 1986) but these rates appear to be rising (Hepworth, 2004). The disorder has been analysed from several perspectives. The most long standing and arguably the most powerful of these perspectives is the medical or psychiatric perspective. This centres on appetite restriction and weight loss, and identifies precursors to anorexia such as weight phobia and a need for control (see Chapters 1 and 4). As well as emphasising physiological issues, psychiatric accounts may also encompass broader social and feminist explanations (see Chapters 1 and 4). Thus, even in biomedicine there is a relatively diverse range of dimensions around which the illness is discussed. This diversity is increased when sociological explanations (usually feminist) are considered.

Some early feminist work (e.g. Chernin, 1986) was written by women who themselves had experienced an eating disorder. The work of these writers 'constituted a series of first moves by feminists working around AN' (Hepworth, 2004:371). Feminists have frequently described anorexia as an unconscious social protest against the constraints and contradictions of women's lives. (Orbach, 1993). Self-starvation, in Orbach's view, is a political act. In describing the anorectic's behaviour, Orbach suggests:

> Like the hunger striker, she has taken as her weapon a refusal to eat. Like the suffragettes [...] she is giving urgent voice to her protest. The hunger strike becomes the means of protest to draw attention to [...] the moral righteousness of the cause [...] the necessity for action. (Orbach, 1993:83)

Orbach uses the image of political struggle as a social metaphor for anorexic behaviour in a patriarchal world. Bordo however, (1988) suggests that the anorexic protest does not take the form of a conscious political battle. Anorexia is a disease, not the active championing of a political cause. Nevertheless in rejecting female sexuality, the anorexic is engaged in a sub-conscious protest against a problematic social role – the restricted, exploited and degraded role of adult femininity. Ironically however, by making herself ill the anorexic is helping to maintain a stereotype of women as neurotic and in need of control.

Katzman and Lee (1997:392) explain that a milieu which 'honours personal power, relational satisfaction and political position in the family and society at large' may help to counteract the social forces which give rise to anorexia. Anorexia is a 'consequence of a mysoginistic society that demeans women by devaluing female experience, by objectifying their bodies and by discrediting areas of women's achievement' (Banks, 1992:873). In developing an eating disorder, the anorexic is challenging the undermining of women's experience in patriarchal society, and is thus engaging in a political resistance. The model of the anorexic as hunger striker (Orbach,

1993), engaged in a struggle against the undervalued role of adult femininity, may therefore be valid.

Some authors, however, have argued that the lack of political consciousness on the part of the pitifully sick anorexic, entirely refutes the 'anorexic as hunger striker' model. In an often quoted passage Brumberg (1988b) remarks, 'if the anorexics' food refusal is political [...] it is a severely limited and infantile form of politics, directed primarily at parents [...] without any [...] allegience to a larger collectivity' (Brumberg, 1988b:37). Whether or not one agrees with this model, it is surely undeniable that a pressure to conform to conflicting roles, and the frustrations of being falsely assured of equal opportunities in what remains essentially a masculinist culture, are factors which contribute to anorexia. The pressures of enforced sexual availability and vocational motherhood, the disenfranchisement and humiliation derived from the objectification of women's bodies which occurs routinely in the media, may all serve to undermine women's self-esteem and drive them into the disorder.

Feminists also argue that women have to function in several different worlds (Katzman and Lee, 1997) such as the public and private worlds of work and the family. Women may use anorexia as a way of addressing the conflicts involved in the transition between these worlds. This implies that women's bodies are inscribed with social significance and may act as a focus on which these conflicts may be acted out. Katzman and Lee (1997) define specifically gendered illness in the late twentieth and early twenty-first century, as resulting from disconnection. Women move from one cultural environment to another often through status changes as a result of the gains of feminism. They may deploy food control as a way of coping with the disconnection they thus experience.

Anorexia as a culture bound syndrome

Anorexia nervosa is thus inseparable from the society in which it arises. As indicated in Chapter 1, definitions of anorexia have developed through an historical process by which 'knowledge' about the illness has become established. We may therefore conclude that the illness comprises a 'Culture Bound Syndrome' (Ritzenbaugh, 1982:347). Culture Bound Syndromes (CBSs) are specific to certain cultures and periods in history. Anorexia may be understood as culture bound as it occurs at a specific point in the history of western capitalist societies. Also, a culture bound syndrome can only be understood inside its cultural context (Ritzenbaugh, 1982). Anorexia conforms to this criterion, as it is based on the social pathologising of fatness characteristic of the West. Furthermore, a disease may be considered culture bound when it summarises the core norms of the culture. Anorexia clearly incorporates the societal valuation of thinness in modern society.

Cecil Helman (1987) analysed the function of culture bound syndromes by invoking the concepts of 'structure' and 'anti-structure'. These describe the instructive and didactic role which illnesses may play for society. In the case of anorexia the accepted normal activities of healthy dieting conform to 'structure', while the distorted, pathological activity of anorexia represents 'anti-structure'. As a disorder, anorexia exemplifies the morbidity of the pursuit of extreme thinness, thus reinforcing the acceptability of sensible dieting which does not go too far. Anorexia therefore is a product of the lifeworld, but also provides a commentary on it. As well as being a distorted and disapproved of form of socially sanctioned behaviour, anorexia is also an enactment of the cultural exhortation to be thin.

Giddens (1991) views anorexia as concerned with the body and the self-project. Giddens feels that the anorexic is in possession of a false self, a self that does not feel at home in the body. The anorexic may not be aware that her (or his) anorexic solution is deeply rooted in the project of the self, but nevertheless 'anorexia represents a striving for security in a world of plural but ambiguous options [...] the tightly controlled body is an emblem of a false existence in an open social environment' (1991:107). Giddens describes anorexic control as 'compulsive mastery' (1991:107), different from healthy reflexivity in that it controls the subject while the latter is controlled by her.

From a post-structuralist perspective, Bordo (1993) argued that women achieve power through dieting and that this was a form of 'disciplinary practice' carried out by individual women on themselves.

In the case of anorexia such activity becomes morbidly obsessive, reflecting the 'heterogeneous distress of our age'. Like Giddens and Bordo, Turner (1996) also views anorexia from the perspective of the sociology of the body. Turner sees anorexia as a product of 'calculated hedonism', a representational disease based wholly on concerns with how the body is represented in society.

Turner also emphasises the following. Firstly anorexia is influenced by the social organisation of life into public and private spheres, and the (slowly) growing representation of women in public. Secondly, anorexia may be understood as a medicalising process whereby women's distress (which should presage political action) is relegated into a passive illness. The medicalising of women's distress is an important issue in analysing anorexia. In constructing anorexia as an illness, biomedicine has re-interpreted in clinical terms the long-term pain which women experience, and has rendered this pain as a chronic disease. As a chronic condition, anorexia has something in common with other chronic conditions and it is thus appropriate to analyse anorexia with reference to sociological writing in other areas of chronic illness. Such and analysis will now be offered.

Anorexia as a Chronic Illness

In applying a sociological analysis to the study of anorexia, the body of work developed by researchers in the field of chronic illness has a significant contribution to make. Chronic Illnesses are long-term, persistent conditions (Kleinman, 1988, Kelly and Field, 1996, Strauss et al, 1984) including conditions such as arthritis (Bury, 1988), back pain, psoriasis (Jobling, 1988) and mental disorders (Goffman, 1963). This chapter applies insights developed in the field of chronic illness to the study of anorexia.

Patients who are chronically ill differ from those who suffer from short-term, acute illnesses. Though painful and incapacitating, such illness is finite, and, (if not terminal) a full recovery may be made.

Chronic illness however lasts for many months or years, and in some cases will persist for the rest of the sufferer's life. Anorexia is a long term condition and some anorexics complain that they never fully feel free of the illness (Lawrence, 1995). Like other chronic patients, anorexics may experience acute episodes, where symptoms become especially severe (Kleinman, 1988). In non-acute phases also, anorexics may be chronically conscious of the underlying disease and the ever-present threat of the re-emergence of symptoms. For this reason it is important to review anorexia with reference to sociological writing in the field of chronic illness.

Locker (2003) explains that chronic illness has two dimensions. One dimension is their physiological (or psychiatric) effect. The other dimension centres on the 'connotations that particular conditions carry' (2003:87). Certain illnesses, therefore, have a certain image and carry a certain stigma (Goffman, 1963). Illnesses such as anorexia, AIDS and leprosy for example, all carry a stigma of a certain kind. The experience of carrying this label, together with the physical alterations in the patient's body which occur as a result of illness, (along with feelings of uncertainty about the future), will often have a serious effect on the way patients see themselves, and the course of their lives. On being diagnosed with anorexia, for example, the patient is forced to confront the reality of having a serious psychiatric illness by which she may be defined for many years. The patient's perception of his or her life course therefore changes in a process Bury refers to as 'biographical disruption' (1982:167). This disruption and change in self concept will be discussed later in this chapter.

Long term disease may therefore give rise to specific experiences, which are common to most forms of chronic illness. These experiences are shared by the chronically ill, including anorexics. Such experiences include the challenge of managing symptoms, stigma and changes in self-concept. Each of these areas will be addressed in this chapter, which will outline the similarities between anorexia and other forms of chronic illness. The first of these areas, the practicalities of managing the illness, will now be discussed.

The practicalities of managing the illness

I will begin this appraisal of the similarities between anorexia and other forms of chronic illness with an account of the practical difficulties anorexics face in the daily management of their symptoms. Most anorexics are treated on an outpatient basis where they manage many of their symptoms at home. This 'home management' experience is shared by many other sufferers of chronic illnesses (Radley, 1994) and may result in disruption and social isolation. Strauss et al (1984) highlight the isolation generated by embarrassment over symptoms and the 'daily grind' of illness management which often results in limited contact with others. Chronically ill patients, including anorexics, may thus become socially isolated and may feel more in common with fellow sufferers than with other members of society.

Scambler (2003b) argues that the vast majority of care for chronically ill people is provided by families, and this may also be the case for anorexics. Parents, partners or spouses may be asked to provide support and care and to ensure that the sufferer is eating. Family support cannot be taken for granted however, and, as Bury explains (1988) 'there is no guarantee that significant others will respond in a wholly predictable or supportive manner' (1988:92), particularly in view of the long term nature of the disorder. As a result, anorexics and other chronically ill patients, may find themselves relying on community care provided by the NHS.

Many chronic patients, including anorexics, find their employment status and career prospects alter (Locker, 2003), perhaps even with the loss of their job. Strauss et al (1984) refers to this experience as the 'pauperizaton process' when the sufferer is forced 'to give up an otherwise satisfactory career' (Strauss et al, 1984:13). The loss of a key role (i.e. worker) which chronic illness often presages may lower self-esteem and alter the sufferer's sense of his or her identity (Locker, 2003, Bury,1988) and the hospitalised anorexic is not excepted from this process. Out-patient anorexics, however, may differ in this regard from other anorexics. For anorexic out-patients, increased activity (including exercise and academic work) may be part of their symptoms. Maintaining role efficiency thus may be less problematic for these anorexics than for other chronic illness patients. Thus 'the need to resolve the compelling demands of bodily symptoms and those of society' (Radley, 1994:152) which most chronic patients experience, may press less heavily. If she eventually becomes an in-patient, however the anorexic may experience a similar degree of pauperisation to other chronic patients.

Loss of self identity

On first being diagnosed, chronically ill patients often experience a huge sense shock (McDonald, 1988, Locker 2003, Bury, 1988). Anorexics, especially those who retain the classic 'anorexic delusions' of having normal eating patterns and being of normal weight, may thus be distressed by their diagnosis and may have to make the adjustment from a normal self image to a 'psychiatrically disordered' identity. On being diagnosed, anorexics may have to re-construct themselves as 'mentally unbalanced' and in need of psychiatric care. Like other mentally ill patients, their identity is thus radically changed as they move towards acknowledging their 'impaired' mentally ill status.

The reconstruction of self-image is therefore a central feature in chronic illness (Locker, 2003). Kelly and Field (1996) argue that a key component in the sufferer's changing self image lies in the manner in which the individual perceives their own body. 'The building up of the self comes from outside through the investiture of social meanings' derived from the appearance of the body. 'Core identities such as gender age and ethnicity are typically embodied [...] Many [...] identities are "read off" and imputed by others on the basis of physical appearance' Kelly and Field (1996:243). The emaciated appearance of the anorexic may cause others to attribute a certain identity (e.g. 'unbalanced') to the sufferer which may in turn impact on the sufferer's view of themselves. It is often argued that in the initial stages of anorexia, patients adopt the disorder as a manner of establishing a self-identity in order to assert a degree of independence and control (Bruch, 1978, Orbach, 1993, Lawrence, 1995, MacSween, 1993). This might imply that far from being damaging to the sufferer's sense of self, anorexia actually enhances it. The self-identity established by the anorexic through extreme thinness and rigid control of food, is however, a very shaky identity dependent on ever increasing food restriction, and constantly threatened by the demand of overwhelming appetite. Also, once diagnosed, the sufferer is forced to confront the possibility that she has a serious psychiatric illness, and such realisation may damage her sense of self and her view of the course of her life just as other chronic illness does.

Williams (1984) explains how chronic illness 'may [thus] assault an individual's sense of identity' (175). This may lead the sufferer to search for meaning in explaining the onset of their illness. Such meaning may take a religious form (e.g. as illness as retribution for past sins), or may constitute a 'scientific' reflection on possible social or environmental causes for the illness (such as bereavement or work stress). Either way, such a search for meaning allows the patient to understand the illness in the context of his or her biography and to re-establish an inner sense of confidence that the life course goes on. The reasons patients use to account for their illness constitute reference points which allow the patient to make sense of her or his experience. Such reference points may be constructed by anorexics who may explain their illness by referring to serious life events such as bereavement (see Chapter 7). By reconstructing their biography in this way, anorexics, and other chronic illness patients may be attempting to render their experience as explicable or even normal. Such a strategy may help to offset another key effect of chronic illness, which is the experience of stigma. A discussion of the issue of stigma will now be presented.

Stigma

A key issue identified by researchers in the field of chronic illness is the concept of stigma. As Bury points out 'different conditions carry with them different connotations and images' (1991: 453). AIDS patients, for example may be constructed as promiscuous, and blind people as possessing 'gravity of thought'. Stigma thus results from the socially constructed characteristics associated with specific illnesses. Today the especially stigmatised illnesses include AIDS, herpes and cancer (Klienman, 1988). Anorexia carries the stigma of being puzzling and threatening – a long-term condition with very serious consequences. Just as for other chronic illness, the meaning of anorexia therefore derives from the cultural construction of what constitutes an anorexic. Constructed as ghoulish and baffling, an illness such as anorexia may greatly influence the way in which a sufferer sees her or himself once they have been diagnosed, and also may affect how others see the sufferer. In this way, myths surrounding the illness become 'the established script for ritual behaviour' applied to the affliction (Kleinman, 1988:26).

Stigmatised illness, once diagnosed, may therefore have detrimental social effects on the lives of sufferers. The attitude of others to the stigmatised may be dominated by their perceptions of the illness which then acquires 'master status' (Scambler, 2003b) overwriting other elements of the person's identity (Kelly and Field, 1966). Stigma is often to do with what is physically visible, (e.g. emaciation in anorexia). These 'external signals deriving from the disease' are key social symbols by which sufferers are singled out from the 'normal' population. This may be especially the case for anorexics who are stigmatised as freakish and unfathomable. As Kleinman (1988) explains:

> [Stigma is] the carapace of culturally marked illnes, a dominant societal symbol that, once applied to a person, spoils radically that individual's identity and is not easily removed [...] cultural meanings mark the sick person, stamping him or her with significance often unwanted, and neither easily warned off nor coped with. (1988:22–6)

Discredited and discreditable

The chronically ill may feel a need to conceal their condition from others. Anorexics may also wish to conceal their illness, and in this regard have much in common with other chronic illness sufferers such as AIDS patients (Simoni and Ng, 2002). If the illness were to become public knowledge, the patient in Goffman's words becomes 'discredited' (1963:3). Even where it is possible to conceal the illness, the patient remains potentially discreditable, permanently at risk of exposure. In either case the illness is 'internalized as a "spoiled identity", a feeling of being inferior, degraded, deviant and shamefully different' (1963:3).

The stigmatised person is thus alien and those who share a specific illness may also share a specific stigma. Thus they will experience similar changes in their self-images and a similar 'moral career' (Goffman, 1963, Kleinman, 1988). Although patients may reject this discredited identity 'either way their world has been radically altered' (Kleinman, 1988:160).

Scambler (2003b) discusses stigmatisation from the perspective of 'labeling' theory. He identifies the issue of 'primary' and 'secondary' deviance in the labeling process. Primary deviance describes the experience of becoming ill. Secondary deviance is the effect on the recipient of being labeled as ill. Often the effects of labeling an ill patient may be far more damaging than their physiological experience of illness. Scambler and Hopkins (1986), for example, describe the process by which epileptic patients felt they had been 'made into epileptics', as a result of the physician 'outing' them through his diagnosis. Thus when doctors apply labels to patients they are wielding considerable power. This power to define and diagnose disease can profoundly affect the lives and identities of patients and for this reason it is important to discuss the process by which chronic illness labels are constructed and applied. Such a discussion is offered in the next section.

Application of Chronic Illness labels

Doctors are charged with assigning labels to illness. They also take responsibility for defining labels which are collectively used to define diagnoses (Locker, 2003). These collective definitions of disease are then applied to patient's accounts in the illness consultation when the doctor selects those aspects of the 'history' which indicate that the patient is suffering specific clinical symptoms. The clinical definition of the patient's illness is then given priority over the patient's account. The patient's broader view of her illness (which may encompass a wider view of causes (such as work stress or bereavement) and effects (e.g. on employment or self-esteem) may thus be ignored.

Several sociologists have attempted to theorise the construction of illness categories in the interaction between patients and doctors (Freidson, 1970a, Nettleton, 1995, Mishler, 1984, Weitz, 2001, Helman, 2000, Bury, 1982, Kelly and Field, 1996). These researchers have argued that doctors and patients view illness in different ways. To the doctor, illnesses are specific syndromes with a series of symptom manifestations. Using scientific 'knowledge' the doctor reviews these symptoms to assess if the patient has a specific syndrome. The doctor thus normally applies a 'scientific' model to assessing disease. The patient however may have a very different understanding of her illness, which incorporates its effects (such as job loss and the impact on her family) and the personal context in which her illness has occurred. Thus the patient understands her illness using a 'lay' explanatory model.

In the clinical consultation the scientific model and the lay model combine, in a process where illness appraisal is negotiated between the patient and the doctor (Freidson, 1970a, Nettleton, 1995, Mishler, 1984, Weitz, 2001, Helman, 2000). Usually however, because of his/her position of authority, the doctor's model of the illness prevails. Scientific knowledge is therefore privileged over lay understandings (Weitz, 2001, Fisher, 2001, Lupton, 1994) and patients' 'lay' accounts often fail to emerge.

When the patient visits the doctor, lay and clinical models will interact. In addition doctors will bring their own lay understandings to the illness consultation (Helman, 2000), while patients also may have some technical knowledge (Fisher, 2001). As a result, lay and clinical models may not always be distinct. In general, however, doctors adopt a technical-scientific view while patients adopt a 'common sense' approach (Mishler, 1984). Because of the professional and social authority they enjoy, doctors are usually in a more powerful position than patients in the clinical consultation. They may be primed to focus on particular manifestations of the disorder at the expense of others.

Doctors may thus interpret patients' accounts to fit the pre-defined criteria they are looking for. A full account of the patient's experience may therefore not emerge, since doctors may subordinate the patient's account to their own bio-technical paradigm.

This focus on the technical aspects of the patient's problem may mean that when the anorexic expresses distress and is perplexed about the causes of her illness, the doctor may largely ignore her distress and continue to check for specific physical symptoms, such as weight loss. In this way, the patient's 'lifeworld' (Mishler, 1984) is subsumed into the psychiatrist's technical-rational system. This process does not simply amount to the doctor imposing his or her view of the world onto the patient however. As Fisher explains:

> The issue here is not that the patient has no power or that the doctor has all of the power. Patients can seek second opinions or change doctors. They can and do ask questions, interrupt, change topics and claim and/or maintain the floor. Doctor's styles of communication can and do vary – some being more dominant and others more egalitarian [but even though] doctors' styles can vary and patients can have input into the decision making process, the asymmetry of the medical relationship remains constant. This institutional authority of the medical role and the control it provides for the physician does not change. (2001:60–74)

As early as 1970, therefore, Freidson explained that in the field of medicine, power rests with the clinician. In 'the modern world' Freidson, explains, 'it is medicine's view of illness that is officially sanctioned and on occasion administratively imposed' (1970a:206). In assessing the patient, the doctor re-frames the patient's problems as technical so as to 'arrive at a specific diagnosis' (Mishler, 1984:10). Jobling (1988) therfore suggests that chronically ill patients 'have a given organisation of experience and even manifestation of the illness, imposed upon them' (1988: 229).

Freidson (1970a) and Fisher (2001) emphasised the importance of language in constructing illness in a specific form. Scientific language may have a positive role in this regard by providing 'benchmarks against which the experience may be evaluated' (Kelly and Field, 1996:242). At the same time, however, the technical language deployed by the doctor signals institutional authority and the institutional power vested in the doctor is 'reflected in the way language is used' (Fisher, 2001:165). This language is applied both in the 'interpersonal' setting of the doctor /patient interview, as well as at the wider social level of disease classification and health education. 'Illness' therefore 'has particular meanings for practitioners who listen to the patient's account [...] in light of their own special interest'.

Kleinman therefore suggests that the bio-technical approach described above may be inappropriate in the management of chronic illness.

> a rigidly bio-medical approach to acute disease for which magic bullets can provide cures [...] essential to using the right magic bullet, is often appropriate and effective. Even for acute exacerbations of chronic disorders, where life threatening biological problems must be controlled, it has its place. But it is inappropriate in the care of chronic illness [...] this biomedical professional model [...] is a reflection of a particular set of values about the nature of the disorder, the work of medicine and the nature of human beings that is frankly destructive in the care of the chronically ill. (1988:136)

This is because, by failing to attend to the patient's own account of the reasons for the worsening of their symptoms, (such as work stress or bereavement) doctors may bewilder, upset and frustrate patients thus adding to, rather than lessening their problems (Kleinman, 1988).

> The message the practitioner indirectly transmits to patients is this 'Your view doesn't really matter much' [...] This medicocentric view is increasingly at odds with the kind of care patients and families want and today expect for chronic illness. (Kleinman: 1988:130)

Kleinman thus argues that doctors should be 'self-reflective interpreters of distinctive systems of meaning' (1988:17).

Doctors' 'interpretive schemes' are 'portmanteau filled with personal and cultural biases' creating 'invidious stereotypes (e.g. "your typical pain patient")' (Kleinman, 1988:53). Looking for 'hard', 'real' diseases, doctors may consider chronic illness as annoying and untidy, and the human stories which accompany it as none of their concern. Like Kleinman, Strauss et al (1984:7) also criticise the 'categorical' approach of medicine as omitting the most important considerations (namely social) in chronic illness. While accepting the usefulness of mainstream biomedical procedures, Strauss et al emphasise the importance of supplementing this with information from the patient's everyday existence.

To gain control, patients may want to find explanations that make sense and allow them to put their condition into perspective. According to Bury (1982) neither patient nor doctor has complete knowledge so should pool their expertise. Williams (1984) concurs that narratives 'are necessarily co-authored' (181), while 'the medical gaze', Locker (2003) argues 'is frequently a narrow one' (Locker, 2003:90). Locker suggests that physicians may lack knowledge about chronic conditions given the complex nature of these illnesses, and given that hospitals generally cater for acute rather than chronic disorder. A more inclusive approach , which takes the patient's as well as the clinician's perspective into account is therefore required.

Conclusion

This review of current sociological literature in the study of anorexia concluded with a discussion of anorexia as a chronic illness. It began however, by discussing the profound social significance which food has to the anorexic in structuring her own life, and more particularly, to the structuring of social life in general. The review then discussed the social significance of eating, particularly with regard to the way in which women eat differently to men in order to achieve a socially valued body. To this end, women diet and a discussion of dieting was therefore presented. Since women diet to alter the shape of their bodies, the sociology of the body was subsequently briefly discussed, and the current social pre-occupation with body perfection described. When the exercise and dieting thus involved becomes obsessive, anorexia may ensue and in the second half of the chapter anorexia was discussed in detail. Feminist and sociological insights were described but the disorder was interpreted particularly with reference to research in the field of chronic illness. The chapter explained that, just as with other forms of chronic illness, the process of being diagnosed as anorexic has profound consequences for the sufferer's self identity. This may force the patient to adjust to a compromised self, and to restructure her plans for the future course of her life. In addition, research in the field of chronic illness is concerned with the process by which chronically ill patients are stigmatised and labelled. The manner in which disease labels are generated and applied by doctors is of central relevance to the current text. The generation of ideas about illness structure and cause will later be applied to the data gathered in this study, particularly in relation to the development of stereotypical definitions of anorexia. In this book I thus analyse the way in which the concept of anorexia is defined, and the implications this may have for the sufferer. To capture the experience of a sample of anorexics, the study adopted a specific methodology. A detailed account of this methodology will now be offered.

Chapter 3
Research Methods

The Aim of the Chapter

This book investigates specific aspects of medical knowledge surrounding anorexia. It considers whether medicine constructs a 'stereotype' of the affluent, high achieving anorexic (Bruch, 1973, Morgan and Russell, 1975). Such a stereotype suggests that the anorexic is afraid of fatness and afraid to grow up (Crisp, 1995). The current study aims to evaluate whether this powerful stereotype has evidence to support it, and whether clinical knowledge surrounding anorexia is substantiated by the data collected in this study. This chapter describes the methods deployed to meet these aims.

Initially, the chapter supplies a broad overview of the various elements of the study. The methodological issues associated with the study of eating disorder are presented and the concept of anorexia as a complex, multiply caused phenomenon is discussed. The implications of this complexity for the selection of methods is addressed, followed by a detailed account of the actual design, methods, and instruments used in the study. The first of these areas, an overview of the various parts of the study will now be discussed.

Overview of the Various Parts of the Study

Clinical knowledge surrounding anorexia is highly complex and so also is the process of deconstructing this knowledge. The current study had several components and this chapter begins with a brief overview of each of these. Firstly, I conducted a review of psychiatric research to establish the existence of the stereotype (Chapter 4). Secondly, demographic data (on age, education, residence and social class) were collected from 104 anorexics. Thirdly, the cognitive stereotype, (based on fat phobia and maturity fear), was tested on a sub-set of 24 anorexic patients. Fourthly, an open-ended interview was conducted (by a doctor) on the same sub-set of 24. The data collected in the study are summarised below:

Table 3.1: Data Collected in the Study

Type of data collected	Number of respondents	
Demographic data only	80	
Demographic data Closed-ended data on fat phobia and maturity fear Narrative interview	24	} = 104

Each of these data were collected to examine the nature of the cognitive and demographic stereotype of anorexia. The chief focus of the study was therefore on cognitive and demographic issues. A further issue however also emerged during the course of the study. Patients often used clinical jargon (such as 'obsessive-compulsive disorder') to describe their illness. I hypothesised that patients may have acquired this vocabulary from clinicians and from the media. I therefore investigated the extent to which this jargon was used and whether patients had 'picked up' this jargon from clinicians. The series of 24 doctor-patient interviews were thus examined to assess whether the doctor 'steered' the patient towards conceptualising her disorder in clinical terms.

The Link between the Aims of the Study and Study Design and Methods

This chapter will indicate that the data gathered in the study and the procedures by which these data were collected were appropriate for testing the study's hypothesis, namely that clinical knowledge surrounding anorexia may not always be supported by data. The study was designed to be sufficiently rigorous to ensure it accessed appropriate dimensions by which its hypothesis could be tested. In particular, data was gathered from acute anorexic patients. Previous sociological studies of anorexia (e.g. MacSween, 1993) have focused on non-acute cases where anorexia was manifested in comparatively mild form. By focussing on acute cases, (manifesting the phenomenon of interest intensely), the current study has uncovered important phenomena which previous studies may have missed.

Acutely ill patients are in a 'dangerous' phase of their disorder. It was therefore essential that the open-ended interviews were conducted by a psychiatrist, to ensure that painful issues were immediately dealt with in a therapeutic manner. I thus secured the services of a specialist registrar from a mental health unit to interview the patients. This doctor was in no way involved with the treatment of the patients whose only contact with her was for the purposes of the study.

The doctor/patient interview formed a key focus of the study, by enabling me to access detailed narrative information on the rich and multi-causal nature of anorexia. The multi-causal nature of the illness was central to the methods selected and an appraisal of this issue will now be offered.

The Multi-Causal Nature of Anorexia

Several researchers have suggested that health research should be conducted within a framework of multi-causality (Burns and Grove, 1993, Palmer, 1989, Lupton, 1994, Prince, 1985). If one accepts that eating disorders are multiply caused manifestations of weight preoccupation, one might also suppose that they could be usefully investigated using a range of different research approaches. Such a strategy is referred to as triangulation. (Zelditch, 1962, Denzin, 1970, 1989).

Denzin (1970, 1989) described four types of triangulation. The first of these is data triangulation, which involves the collection of data from multiple sources in the same study. In a study of domestic labour, for example, data triangulation might involve interviewing wives and husbands to gather information from two independent sources. The second form of triangulation is investigator triangulation. This involves the use of more than one investigator (e.g. two academic colleagues) in the same study. Both investigators could then compare their data to validate the study's findings. A third form of triangulation, theory triangulation is also used. This applies multiple theories to the same data. A study of housework, for example, might be interpreted using both Marxist and feminist theory.[1] Denzin (1970) also describes a fourth type of triangulation, methodological triangulation. This involves the use of more than one research method in the same study. For example, two different types of data collection technique, (such as a quantitative questionnaire and a qualitative interview), might be used.

While useful for validating data, the idea that triangulation can be applied to produce a gradually unfolding picture may be misleading (Silverman, 2000). Triangulation may instead make the picture more complicated, thus obscuring key messages. When applied judiciously, however, triangulation can illuminate aspects of the phenomenon under investigation. In the current study methodological triangulation

1 Marxists would stress housework's contribution to capitalism, while feminists would emphasise its equal contribution to patriarchy (Malos, 1980).

was applied. Two different types of data were collected – open-ended narrative data on the causes of anorexia, along with closed-ended data on age, social class, education and place of residence. In addition, further closed-ended data on anorexic symptoms (see Appendix) were also collected.

The Data Gathering Instruments 1: The Quantitative Questionnaires

The demographic questionnaire

The first questionnaire to be administered was the demographic questionnaire. This investigated the patient's age, sex, class, educational attainment and place of residence. The demographic questionnaire was administered to all 104 anorexics in the study. Patients found this questionnaire easy to complete and only 9 patients omitted to supply information on one or more variables.

1991 census data

Since demographic data formed an important part of the study, it was important to compare this data against similar data for the general population. The most rigorously collected data which could be used for this purpose was census data (OPCS, 1993, 1997) and data from the Department of Education (1996, 2000). Such data were therefore used as a control for data from the sample of 104 anorexics. At the time of the study the 1991 census data were the latest data available and also provided a convenient mid-point comparison between the recruitment of the first anorexic subject (1985) and the last (2001).[2]

2 See page 77.

The EDI-A questionnaire

The second questionnaire to be administered was the 'Eating Disorders Inventory ("Adapted")', (EDI-A, see Appendix and Table 3.2). The EDI is one of the most important and frequently cited screening instruments for anorexia.[3] Its adaptation for the current study was described in Dignon (2006). I examined whether the EDI-A was able to discriminate between healthy women and anorexics. For this reason, the questionnaire was administered to a sub-set of 24 anorexics and 100 healthy controls (see page 76). All found the questionnaire easy to complete, and response rates for all variables were excellent.

Table 3.2: Examples of EDI-A questions

	Always	Usually	Often	Sometimes	Rarely	Never
I am terrified of gaining weight	( )	( )	( )	( )	( )	( )
I wish I could return to the security of childhood	( )	( )	( )	( )	( )	( )

3 Citations by other authors as at 21.4.05: n = 1282 (source: ISI 'World of Knowledge' database).

Potential Bias in the Quantitative Questionnaires

Potential sources of bias inherent in quantitative questionnaires have frequently been identified (Bowling, 1997, Polit and Hungler, 1997). These include 'acquiescence response' which describes the tendency of the subject to endorse rather than disagree with a statement, and 'evaluation apprehension' which describes the anxiety generated in people by virtue of their being assessed. Both sources of bias tend to produce false positives, where, in order to please the researcher, participants present themselves as exhibiting specific attributes which they may not necessarily possess. In the current study, this bias was addressed via the use of pre-validated questionnaires (Garner et al, 1983b, Palmer et al, 1990), and through the use of a census data and a control group. Such bias however represents random error, and is impossible to completely eradicate.

The Data Gathering Instruments 2: The Qualitative Interview

A qualitative interview was administered to 24 of the anorexic patients. The interview aimed to allow patients to discuss in their own words what they felt had caused their illness. Prior to this interview, patients were given the EDI-A (see Appendix). It was hoped that this would induce a process of introspection whereby patients would reflect on the causes of their disorder, and would be more ready to talk about these in a subsequent interview with the doctor. After completing this questionnaire, patients were presented with a very general question:

> What would you say were the causes of your anorexia?

The doctor was asked to allow patients as much time as they needed to answer this question. The conversation which followed, it was envisaged, would take the whole of the interview. If the patient 'dried up' the doctor was asked to maintain the dialogue by referring to general sociological 'causes', such as media influence and the influence of friends and family on attitudes to slimming. This led the doctor to ask questions like 'So you feel your anorexia stemmed from being large as a child?' The interviewer was very careful to keep such prompting to a minimum, but such 'stimulus' questions were nevertheless asked. The interviews were tape recorded, and lasted on average for 25 minutes.

Potential Bias in the Qualitative Interview

The doctor as interviewer

A specialist registrar at a district general hospital conducted the interviews. This doctor was a practising psychiatrist who became involved in the study because she wanted to gain further experience with acutely anorexic patients. Such acute anorexics are somewhat of a rarity, and the study presented the doctor with the opportunity of increasing her knowledge. The doctor was highly experienced and friendly, with a particularly empathic manner. She was referred to the study, to allow her to gain the specialised experience she desired.

It is important however to address problems which may arise as a result of 'second hand' interviewing. These fall under two areas. Firstly the doctor's non-sociological focus may have been inappropriate for this study. Secondly, as a result of the doctor's clinical authority, repondents might have supplied answers they felt the doctor wanted to hear (Lofland and Lofland, 1995). I will deal with each of these issues in turn.

Firstly, the doctor's clinical focus might not have been consistent with the sociological approach. Clinical consultations often result in a short interview (Pope and Mays, 2000). The technique valued by sociologists, conversely, centres on listening, 'remembering what people have said', and achieving 'a good balance between talking and listening' (Mason, 2003:75). Such a model may not be consistent with the speedy, target focused clinical consultation. It is entirely consistent however with the therapeutic technique used by some doctors, particularly psychiatrists. As Pope and Mays explain 'experienced doctors may feel that they already possess [interview] skills and indeed many are transferable' (2000:15). In the current study, the doctor was highly supportive of participants and displayed all the skills characteristic of good interview technique (Mason, 2003, Silverman, 2004). Her non-sociological focus therefore presented very few problems.

The second issue, that of the patient 'clinicalising' her answers (because she was talking to a doctor), is more significant. 'All qualitative interviewers need to consider how they are perceived by interviewees [especially] if the interviewee knows that the interviewer is also a doctor or nurse' (Pope and Mays, 2000:15). At the time of the study, all participants were resident in a psychiatric hospital and were undergoing therapy. The doctor's professional standing may thus have influenced the type of answers given, which might have been expressed in a more 'medicalised' manner.

When patients fashion their answers in a particular way, the interview becomes a forum where facts are constructed, rather than excavated. Such a process however occurs in any research interview. Regardless of the profession of the interviewer, responses are constructed in the context of the interaction (Dey, 1993, Silverman, 2004, Pope and Mays, 2000). Interviews are social encounters where meanings are made anew in the interplay between participant and researcher. Such 'distortion' however, was of interest to the current study. The manner in which patients clinically constructed their answers was part of the study's focus (see Chapter 8). The term 'distortion' may therefore be inappropriate, since the bias produced was central to the research.

Even though this form of bias was of interest however, it was nevertheless important to ensure that patients were interviewed in a standard fashion. Interviews are designed to be open and responsive but in order to uncover the phenomena of interest the interviewer must nevertheless stick to certain topics. In the current study, standardisation was maintained in the following way. Firstly, prior to the interview, I met the interviewing doctor. We agreed that every effort should be made to ensure that questions were as consistent as possible. It was decided that the interviewer would act as a facilitator to bring the patients' feelings to the fore. At the same time I was careful not to minimise the doctor's natural discourse and the very biases which were the focus of the study. The 'biases' inherent in natural discourse therefore emerged (see Chapter 8), and could be observed all the more validly given my efforts to control them.

Recruitment of the EDI-A Control Group

As well as recruiting a sample of anorexics (Box 1), the study also recruited a convenience sample of 100 healthy women. These women were recruited as a control group against which responses from anorexics on EDI-A items could be compared. I recruited these women in the Town Hall Gardens in a city centre in 1997. The Town Hall Gardens is a green area, where large numbers of people come to relax in fine weather. It was chosen as a recruiting site, since it was convenient area in which to approach seated people. I recruited the controls over a six-week period and asked them to complete the EDI-A (see Appendix). The control sample were mostly young, but for the sake of balance, some 'older' women (> 40, n = 9, > 30, n = 14) were also recruited. The ages of participants were guessed by the researcher (prior to approaching a subject), and were later recorded on the questionnaire. No male controls were recruited, but 3 of the sample of 104 anorexics were male.

The nature of the project was explained to each control participant. Permission was then sought to include her in the study, and participants were asked if they had ever experienced an eating

Box 1: How patients were recruited to the study

1. Permission to conduct the study was gained from the Director of the Eating Disorders Unit (EDU) and the Research Ethics Committee

2. The study analysed information from 104 anorexic patients. Twenty four were recruited between 1996 and 2001. Eighty were recruited between 1985 and 1990.

3. For 24 of the anorexic patients (recruited between 1996 and 2001), the Specialist Registrar working on the study approached the patient's key worker (a nurse) and asked for permission to recruit the patient. All anorexic in-patients were approached.

4. The nature of the study was explained to the patient. She was then given an information and consent form.

5. Of 26 patients asked, 24 agreed to participate. Those who declined did so without supplying a reason. An interview appointment was made for those who agreed to take part.

6. The interview was conducted in the standard interview room, in a mental health unit. The room was pleasantly furnished with a homely decor. Patients were dressed in their ordinary day clothes (rather than in pyjamas or a dressing gown), and the doctor was also dressed in ordinary clothes. The doctor did not wear a white coat and no clinical paraphernalia (such as a stethoscope) were visible.

7. The interviewer was experienced in applying empathic techniques in therapeutic consultations. Patients were approached in a sensitive way, and any painful issues that were raised in the interview were immediately explored in a therapeutic manner. The interviewer was in no way involved with the clinical management of the patient whose only contact with her was for the purposes of the study.

disorder.[4] They then completeted the EDI-A (which took roughly 15 minutes). Participants found the questionnaire easy and nobody omitted any of the questions. One hundred and ten women were approached, eight of whom refused to participate because of lack of time. Two people refused without supplying a reason.

The Study Sample – Qualitative Data

For the 24 patients recruited between 1996–2001 (from whom qualitative data were collected), the study employed a purposive sampling design, where patients were selected according to their ability to supply information about anorexia. Acute patients were considered highly information rich (Polit and Hungler, 1997) and such patients were thus recruited. Each patient was diagnosed as suffering from anorexia according to DSM-III or IV criteria (APA, 1980, 1994).

Analysis of the Data

Data from the quantitative questionnaires

Data from the quantitative questionnaires were entered onto SPSS version 9 (Foster, 2001). There were two quantitative questionnaires. The first collected demographic information, the second information from the EDI-A (see Appendix). From the demographic information, frequency tables were produced and chi-square tests were used to test for levels of agreement between anorexic and census data.

The EDI-A measured cognitive symptoms such as fear of fatness and fear of maturity. An EDI-A score was produced, from both the

4 No participant answered yes to this enquiry.

anorexics and the control subjects. This was achieved by adding the number of positive responses to each question. A cut off point of 20 was applied, meaning that participants had to affirm two thirds of the questions to be deemed to have met EDI criteria. This was a slightly higher cut-off point than normally used in the full EDI.[5]

Data from the qualitative interview

The data from the qualitative interviews were interpreted using thematic analysis (Hewitt-Taylor, 2001). Taped interviews were fully transcribed and these transcripts were then coded into themes using the NUD.IST qualitative data analysis package (Gahan and Hannibal, 1998). Themes such as 'unhappiness' and 'control' were extracted from patient narratives, which were then coded into categories. These categories were then used to build a theory (see Chapter 7).

A second theory describing the medicalisation of patients' accounts was also developed. This was based on data which indicated that patients used medical terms to describe their condition. Clinical 'biases' formed a key focus of the theory and were the chief process around which this theory was built (see Chapter 8).

Conclusion

This chapter has outlined the methodology used in the study. It has given an account of data collection methods and has described the data gathering instruments; the management of the open ended inter-

5 It was felt that since the adapted schedule contained fewer questions than the original, it was important that particpants affirmed a higher proportion of these items to meet EDI rating criteria. In any case patient's scores on the global EDI score were a secondary focus of the study, which was more concerned with scores for individual EDI items 'fear of maturity' and 'fear of fatness' (see Chapter 6).

view; the sampling procedure and the subsequent analysis of data. Such an account has made the operational basis of the study transparent. In so doing, it will allow the design of the study to be replicated in future research.

The selection of such design and methods created opportunities for accessing specific information about anorexia. The open ended interview for example, enabled me to compare the meanings attached to anorexia by patients to the narrower clinical stereotype of the illness projected in psychiatric literature and encapsulated in the EDI. This interview also allowed me to examine the extent to which patients had 'medicalised' their accounts of anorexia (see Chapter 8). In addition, the gathering of demographic data allowed me to compare such data against stereotypical definitions of the demographic profile of the 'typical' anorexic patient. Such methodology however also contained limitations. It would have been useful to administer the EDI-A to all 104 anorexics, but the retrospective nature of much of the study design prevented this. In general however the study methodology presented a highly useful opportunity to examine the applicability of 'stereotypical' clinical knowledge to a sample of anorexic patients. In the subsequent five chapters, the study results are presented. The next chapter presents a summary of existing psychiatric research in order to describe the nature of the clinical model of anorexia. These psychiatric studies comprise the vast majority of empirical research into anorexia, and their insights deserve serious consideration. Such consideration is given in the next chapter.

Chapter 4
The Psychiatric Model of Anorexia

Introduction

In this chapter, psychiatric knowledge surrounding anorexia is discussed. The chapter argues that such knowledge may reflect a 'stereotypical' view of anorexia. Initially, the chapter offers an account of the 'mainstream' psychiatric approach, known as family theory. This approach, the chapter argues, theorises anorexia at an individual rather than a social level. The symptom profile that psychiatrists associate with anorexia is then discussed, followed by an account of the limitations of psychiatry, particularly its failure to discuss societal contributors to anorexia. Some psychiatrists have investigated social-cultural factors, however, and the work of these 'socio-cultural' scholars is appraised next. The typical demographic profile assigned to the anorexic by these researchers is identified, and the chapter argues that this profile constitutes a demographic stereotype of the anorexic as a young, bright, middle class city dweller. The limitations of the socio-cultural approach are then summarised, and the chapter explains that some of these limitations have been addressed by feminist psychiatrists. Nevertheless, 'psychiatric' feminism also contains limitations and these are discussed in the subsequent section. A description of psychiatric research that challenges the stereotype then follows, and finally the changing nature of the clinical model is discussed. Such changes are illustrated with reference to the content of medical texts. Most texts reviewed in this chapter were retrieved from databases, so it is important at the outset to describe the search strategy adopted.

The Literature Search

To select appropriate books and articles for review in the current chapter, it was necessary to search appropriate databases. The Psychinfo database was selected as this contains the largest selection of any database of peer reviewed journals and textbooks in psychology and psychiatry. I limited my search to English language articles and books published in the last 30 years, and entered the keywords below:

Keywords	Number of Hits
Anorexia and Weight phobia	22 hits
Anorexia and Obsessionalism	0 hits
Anorexia and Fear of maturity	3 hits
Anorexia and Age	1191 hits
Anorexia and Social class	41 hits
Anorexia and Place of residence	3 hits
Anorexia and Education	227 hits
Anorexia and Feminism	63 hits

As the search yielded hundreds of hits, I used the ISI 'Web of Knowledge' database cited reference search to check which references had been most frequently cited by other authors, and included these in my review. In reading these books and articles, I obtained further references, and I also used my existing knowledge to hand select articles of key relevance. The articles thus obtained covered the 'mainstream' psychiatric approach, the socio-cultural approach, and the feminist-psychiatric approach.

The Psychiatric Approach

Anorexia nervosa is generally viewed as a psychiatric disorder (APA, 1994). The syndrome has been analysed more thoroughly from the standpoint of psychiatry than from any other perspective. The psychiatric approach, which began to emerge in the 1950s and 1960s, is often referred to as 'family theory' (Minuchin et al, 1978, Minuchin, 1991) since family dysfunction and individual pathology are frequently identified as the causes of anorexia (Minuchin et al, 1978, Palmer, 1989). According to the psychiatric approach, the families of anorexics are 'enmeshed' (Minuchin et al, 1978) and isolated from the outside world. They are presented as uncommunicative and lacking in genuine love and spontaneity (Bruch, 1978). Frequently they are characterised as valuing material attainment over genuine displays of love and affection (Bruch, 1978). 'Appearances' and social standing, psychiatrists explain, are what count in these families.

Mothers of anorexics are often characterised by the psychiatric approach as over controlling (Bruch, 1978). They have failed to instil a strong sense of self in their anorexic child, whose subsequent eating disorder is sometimes regarded as a long overdue reaction to a circumscribed environment (Lawrence, 1995). Because of this, psychiatric theories have largely viewed anorexia as a form of rebellion on the part of the sufferer (Crisp, 1995). The anorexic's parents convey high expectations to their adolescent daughters, often as a means of compensating for their own career disappointment (Bruch, 1978). Initially, their daughter becomes a high achiever, but pressures of approaching adulthood and the requirements of independence create an impasse which leads to anorexia.

Psychiatric approaches therefore theorise anorexia in terms of a 'maturational crisis' (Crisp, 1995:63, Palmer, 1989, Bruch, 1978). This crisis is further theorised as a flight from full genital sexuality – a failure to fully adjust to a female adult role. Self-starvation is seen by the anorexic as a way of ridding herself of troublesome womanly curves. Ironically, however, in suppressing her sexuality the anorexic is simultaneously conforming to a male defined idea of slim attractiveness.

According to the psychiatric approach, the anorexic experiences her life as being out of control, (Lawrence, 1995). The demands made by her parents create an overwhelming sense of anxiety. Quite by chance the daughter may go on a diet and successfully lose a few pounds. The exhilaration she derives from this, and her sense of accomplishment and achievement help to assuage anxiety in other areas of her life (Lawrence, 1995). She keeps on dieting to maintain the 'buzz' and gets caught in a downward spiral of ever increasing weight loss and ever more elaborate methods of maintaining food control.

These aspects of the anorexic's behaviour, particularly 'fear of maturity' and the use of food as a strategy of control, have been identified by psychiatrists as typical symptoms of anorexia. As befits a medical approach, psychiatry has expended considerable effort in developing and validating a clinical model of the symptom profile of the 'typical' anorexic. A discussion of this model will now be offered.

Psychiatry's View of the Symptom Profile of the 'Typical' Anorexic

Psychiatrists are trained to apply very strict criteria to the appraisal of anorexia (APA, 1994, APA, 1980). These criteria are usually elicited via the use of closed-ended questionnaires (Garner and Garfinkel, 1979, Garner et al, 1983b) which contain items such as 'fear of maturity'. Often these questionnaires are read out verbatim by the doctor, to ensure that he or she covers the questions in exactly the form laid down in the schedule. A significant portion of the psychiatrist's time is spent learning how to administer psychiatric assessments and in familiarising him or herself with the criteria for a given diagnosis.

Closed-ended diagnostic instruments are widely applied in the research setting (1980). In the clinical setting, the doctor's 'qualitative' clinical judgement is also applied, and so a degree of interpretation of the patient's symptoms is permitted. While this allows for a more fluid assessment, it may also result in the distortion of the patient's symptoms in accordance with the doctor's viewpoint (Lee, 1996). For example, where the patient expresses herself as undervalued and unhappy, the doctor may direct the patient to focus on quantitative details, such as weight loss, in order to 'tick off' diagnostic criteria. One symptom that the patient is always assumed to exhibit is 'fat phobia'. She is restricting her food because she is terrified of becoming fat. Almost all diagnostic manuals therefore construct the disorder as an intense fear of fatness, and subsequent dieting to produce weight loss (Garfinkel, 1992, Russell, 1970, APA, 1994, APA, 1980). In 1970 for example, Russell identified three criteria for anorexia nervosa:

> Behaviour that is designed to produce marked weight loss;
>
> The characteristic psychopathology of becoming fat [i.e. intense fear of fatness];
>
> Evidence of an endocrine disorder – in females, amenorrhea, and in males the loss of sexual potency and interest. (Russell, 1970, cited in Garfinkel, 1992:38)

Other diagnostic criteria have also been specified but all feature aspects of Russell's original rubric (Garfinkel, 1992). What is interesting about these criteria is the extent to which they are rendered in highly physiological terms. For psychiatry, these criteria perform a special function. As well as aiming to uncover the important aspects of anorexic behaviour, they announce by their 'objectivity' that psychiatry is just as scientific as other medical specialisms.

In the criteria identified by Russell, psychiatry demonstrates a somatic focus on bodily concerns. Symptoms such as weight loss and the interruption of the menses (or the sex drive in males), both centre on the physiological effects of appetite restraint. Psychiatry has also focused on psychological as well as somatic symptoms in analysing anorexia. Two of the most important of these symptoms – control and perfectionism/obsessionalism will now be discussed.

Control, Perfectionalism/Obessionalism

In the past fifteen years, psychiatrists have emphasised the importance of anorexia as a strategy of control (Palmer, 1989, Lawrence, 1995). Though absent from clinical classificatory schemes, this criteria has been cited in many textbooks as a contributor to the disorder (Palmer, 1989, Lawrence, 1995). The 'control' criterion argues that the sufferer controls food because she experiences a lack of control in other areas of her life. By embarking on a strict regime of food refusal, the anorexic seeks to re-establish some of the control wrested from her in other spheres. Such loss of control may have occurred as a result of an adverse life event such as sexual abuse (Palmer et al, 1990), or it may simply be the result of stifling parenting in an over-controlling family.

Anorexia has also been analysed as the pursuit of perfectionism (Bruch, 1978, Lawrence, 1995) and obsessionalism (Levenkron, 2000). Lawrence (1995), for example suggests that anorexics have perfectionist personalities. When they succeed at a difficult task they feel better about themselves. This perfectionism is often accompanied by 'obessionalism' (Levenkron, 2000:41), a trait whereby the patient must obsessively perform a certain action (e.g. resisting food), since to do otherwise would produce unbearable anxiety. This perfectionist /obsessionalist dimension has been identified by several researchers (Bruch, 1978, Lawrence, 1984, Strober,1980) as important in the development of anorexia. Along with control, perfectionism forms a key dimension in the Eating Disorders Inventory (Garner et al, 1983b), one of the most important closed-ended psychiatric schedules applied to anorexia. Control and perfectionism must be considered as two of the central symptoms identified by psychiatrists as associated with anorexia.

Limitations of the Psychiatric Approach

The psychiatric approach contains some significant limitations. In diagnosing anorexia, psychiatry rigidly adheres to specific symptomatology. Fat phobia and dieting (and to a lesser extent control, obsessionalism and perfectionism), are privileged as explanations, while other pro-genitors may be invalidated. Psychiatric 'family theory' (Minuchin et al 1978) also contains limitations. It appears to suggest that anorexia derives from a dominant mother imposing control on her daughter. The daughter is raised to achieve success to compensate for her mother's career failure, and is thus caught in a double bind of compliance and competition. The anorexic adopts a strategy of weight control to achieve independence, but is caught in a moral spiral since it is impossible to constantly adhere to her strict regime. She must inevitably fail and feels her failure so deeply that her efforts to lose weight are re-doubled.

The psychiatric approach therefore stigmatises the 'anorexogenic' mother, identifying her as the cause of the disorder. It is this 'mother blaming' approach which is, I feel, the most unhelpful element of the psychiatric paradigm. Such an approach reflects societal assumptions that mothers bear sole responsibility for their children's health and welfare. Lawrence (1995) explains that women are inundated with contradictory advice from experts concerning how this responsibility should be discharged. One minute mothers are told to cuddle a crying baby and feed her on demand, the next minute they are told to feed by the clock and leave a crying baby alone. Such an approach pressurises women and generates anxiety over childcare methods. Psychiatry thus fails to identify the social context in which 'anorexogenic' mothers are located. But psychiatry also fails on another level. Its unswerving emphasis on individual pathology as the cause of the disorder leads it to ignore the importance of society (and the social construction of gender) in creating conditions which lead to anorexia. Existing psychiatric approaches assume that anorexia can be treated at an individual level (using family or behaviour therapy). Such approaches identify maturational crises in anorexic patients, but fail to address the problematic female social identity from which the patient recoils. Instead, they identify the adolescent girl herself as deficient, and attempt to intervene (via therapy) at the level of her psyche. The desired outcome is presumably a 'healthy' individual, fully adjusted to a subordinate social role. MacSween explains:

> [psychiatrists] share in common an individualistic slant which sees anorexia as [...] a problem of individual deviance [...] thus,the culture which produces anorexia is normalized out of their analyses. (1993:51)

Psychiatrists, therefore fail to account for the social and cultural context in which anorexia occurs. By emphasising individual symptomatology and a failure on the part of the anorexic to adjust, psychiatry fails to place the individual's suffering within the context of the wider society. Some psychiatrists however have made an attempt to integrate an appraisal of social issues into their analysis of anorexia nervosa (Crisp et al, 1976, Morgan and Russell, 1975, Azuma and Henmi, 1982, Rathner and Messner, 1993, Hamburg and Herzog, 1985). These psychiatrists are referred to as socio-culturalists.

The Socio-cultural Psychiatric Approach

It may at first seem inappropriate to include a discussion of socio-cultural approaches in a chapter on the psychiatric perspective. It is evident however that almost all research into the link between 'social factors' (such as media, class and education) and anorexia has been conducted by 'socio-cultural' psychiatrists. These researchers have attempted to empirically investigate the influence of society on the development of anorexia. The key findings of socio-culturalists are thus of central interest to sociologists.

The socio-culturalist approach (Boskind-White and White, 1986:353, Garner et al, 1983a:65, Garner and Garfinkel, 1980:647, Toro et al, 1994:147) suggests that social pressures are a measurable component in the analysis of anorexia. Socio-culturalists identify the importance of social institutions (such as the media) in communicating a 'culture of slenderness' (Garner and Garfinkel, 1980:647) to young middle class women (Garner et al, 1983a:65, Garner and Garfinkel, 1980:647, Toro et al, 1994:147). The agencies through which this culture is transmitted are identified (Garner and Garfinkel, 1980), and the importance of sex, class and educational background in the development of anorexia are stressed (see Bruch, 1978, Boskind-White and White, 1986, Crisp et al, 1976, Morgan and Russell, 1975, Hamburg and Herzog, 1985).

In assessing why anorexia affects mainly women, the socio-cultural approach focuses almost entirely on the different social roles assigned to each gender. In particular socio-culturalism describes the concept of gender role adoption (Crisp, 1995, Weeda-Manack, 1994). Anorexics, psychiatrists suggest, are striving to avoid female adulthood, and to halt their development into sexually mature women. While psychiatry acknowledges the differential roles assigned to each sex, it fails to conduct an analysis of why women occupy subordinate status. It has been left to sociologists, such as MacSween (1993), to theorise the mechanisms by which unequal social roles are ascribed (see Chapter 2).

Socio-culturalist findings in relation to Age, Class, Education and Place of Residence

Almost all research into anorexia and its association with age, social class, education, and place of residence has been conducted by socio-culturalists. Their findings suggest that anorexia is pre-dominantly a disorder of the young, urban, educated, middle class (Lucas et al, 1988, Crisp et al, 1976, Hoek and Brook, 1985, Azuma and Henmi, 1982). This research, together with a critique of its methods will now be presented.

The age of the typical anorexic

According to socio-culturalists, anorexics are almost entirely young women. In 1979, for example, Halmi et al discovered that the usual age of onset for anorexia was about 15. Consequently many authors refer to age as a distinguishing feature of anorexia, invariably characterising the anorexic as juvenille. (Bruch, 1978, Rastam et al, 1989, Lucas et al, 1988). Where cases are observed among older women, these women are usually described as having initially developed anorexia in adolescence. Recent evidence suggests however that, in response to life events, anorexia may begin later in life, even during one's 60s or 70s (Wills and Olivieri, 1988). Nevertheless, the picture of the anorexic teenager rejecting full feminine adulthood is one of the most powerful images of the typical anorexic.

The anorexic's social class

Socio-culturalists have traditionally viewed anorexia as a middle class disorder. The experience of being working class according to psychiatrists, seems to have a 'sparing effect' (Crisp et al, 1976). In middle class families, the children are under considerable pressure to maintain the family's standing, by achieving in both the educational and social sphere (Bruch, 1978). At the same time these children are required to be well behaved, obedient and to conform to the rigid control of strict middle class parents. Such an environment, with its limited scope for independence and self-expression, might reasonably be expected to create the conditions in which anorexia may develop.

A significant number of research studies have therefore claimed that anorexia is concentrated in the middle class. This review will focus specifically on four of these studies. Firstly it will describe an investigation conducted by Morgan and Russell in 1975.[1] Secondly, it

1 Citations by other authors as at 21.4.05: n = 467 (source: ISI 'World of Knowledge' database).

will discuss the study conducted by Crisp et al in 1976.[2] Thirdly, the study conducted in 1986 by Szmukler and colleagues[3] will be evaluated, and finally Gower and McMahon's study from 1989 will be appraised.

One of the most widely cited research studies investigating the link between anorexia and social class was conducted by Morgan and Russell in 1975. These researchers recorded the social class background (according to father's occupation) of 41 anorexic patients, and found 'an excess of social class I and II families [66%] (Registrar General's Classification) with a deficiency of social classes III, IV and V' (1975:361). In Morgan and Russell's study, however all subjects had long illness histories. The authors themselves therefore suggested that the presence of these patients in the series, might have reflected 'a willingness to seek psychiatric help' rather than a class bias in the anorexic population. In other words, middle class patients were more likely to seek psychiatric aid and were thus over-represented in the figures. Morgan and Russell's study is nevertheless frequently cited as evidence of anorexia as a middle class disorder.

Crisp et al's (1976) study is also cited as seminal. The study presented the results of the incidence of anorexia in a population of 12,391 students from 2 state and 7 private schools. The authors suggested that anorexia was reasonably common in the private schools (amounting to roughly 1 case in every 100 sixteen-plus aged students), while a far lower incidence (roughly 1 case in every 550 students) was found in the state schools. This led the study to conclude that anorexia is more common among middle class youngsters. Crisp et al's report however has methodological shortcomings. Anorexic cases, for example, were selected thorough the authors' collaboration with teachers. The authors therefore relied on the teachers' awareness of anorexia in order to spot cases of the illness. In a well-funded middle class school it is reasonable to assume that the teachers might strive to

2 Citations by other authors as at 21.4.05: n = 350 (source: ISI 'World of Knowledge' database).

3 Citations by other authors as at 21.4.05: n = 80 (source: ISI 'World of Knowledge' database).

improve their awareness of anorexia. Staff in the state sector may (understandably) have little time for this activity.

Other studies however have reproduced Crisp et al's findings. In 1986, Szmukler et al examined a total of 238 cases of anorexia nervosa on an Aberdeen psychiatric case register, 1965–1982. The authors found an over-representation for classes 1 and II, who between them made up 46% of their sample. Szmukler et al therefore concluded that patients from higher social classes were over-represented in attendance statistics. They further suggested that this trend remained stable over time, invalidating the notion that anorexia is spreading more widely through society. Szmukler et al's study however, has its flaws. Firstly the sample was recruited from patients who had been referred to a specialist clinic. Middle class women (Palmer, 1989) are more likely to be referred to these services are thus over-represented in case registers. Secondly, Szmukler et al's information was recorded from a secondary source of patient records. Some of these records were old and may have contained errors. Notwithstanding, Szmukler et al's study has been widely disseminated as definitive proof that anorexics are predominantly middle class.

A study purporting to show a similar trend was conducted by Gower and McMahon in 1989. Gower and McMahon recorded the socio-economic status of 100 consecutive patients with anorexia nervosa referred to the St Georges Hospital in London. This study observed a marked preponderance (50%) of patients from social classes 1 and 11. The study confirmed, in Gower and McMahon's view, that anorexia remains a middle class disorder. In comparison to other studies of anorexia and class however, the authors conclude that the trend in favour of middle class groups is decreasing. Gower and MacMahon's methods however were deficient. The study provided no control group against which the results from the anorexic sample could be compared, and it was therefore impossible to assess the class distribution of the geographic area from which referrals had been made. If this area was itself middle class, this would have skewed the study's results. Similarly, the issue of referral bias (where middle class women are likely to receive specialist treatment (Palmer, 1989, Gard and Freeman, 1996)), also applies to Gower and MacMahon's study.

In the 1970s and 1980s, four key studies therefore purported to demonstrate that anorexics were largely middle class. Since the 1980s, however, several studies have appeared which identify that anorexia affects women from all socio-economic groups (Whitaker et al, 1989, Lee, 1991, Rogers et al, 1997). Whitaker et al's study , for example, found that dieting behaviour in a community sample of normal weight subjects bore no relationship to the class background of the dieter. Lee observed a similar trend in 1991 where most subjects in his anorectic sample were from lower socio-economic groups. Finally, Rogers and colleague's community survey (1997) found equal levels of clinically significant eating disordered behaviour among working class subjects when compared to their middle class counterparts. According to these studies, therefore the contention that anorexia is a middle class disorder is inaccurate. But this has failed to lead to any general acceptance by clinicians that social classes are evenly distributed within the anorexic population. Doctors appear to persist in their belief that anorexia is predominantly suffered by higher socio-economic groups (Russell, 2000, Gelder et al, 2004).

The anorexic's educational level

As well as describing the anorexic as typically middle class, psychiatric researchers have also suggested that anorexics are usually high educational achievers (Hoek and Brook, 1985). Middle class families, it is suggested, place high expectations on their adolescent daughters to achieve, (Bruch, 1978) and these expectations may be experienced as highly pressuring. In 1985, therefore Hoek and Brook studied the level of educational achievement among 462 anorexics. They compared the anorexics' level of education with that of a control group. A difference in attainment was observed in relation to 'vocational' and 'general' (i.e. academic) education. While 18.9% of the anorexics had an academic education, the figure for the general population was only 3.9%. This would suggest that the anorexics were over four times more likely than their non-anorexic peers to have gained an academic education.

At face value, it may thus appear that anorexics are high achievers. On closer examination however, it is apparent that Hoek and Brook's methodology may have distorted their figures. The authors used all-encompassing categories of vocational and general to describe a highly diverse range of educational qualifications. In deciding which qualification to classify under each label, the researchers used a high degree of interpretation. Also, Hoek and Brook used a retrospective design, by evaluating secondary data in the form of clinical records. Such records are often incomplete, as they were originally gathered to record clinical rather than educational data. Findings from these records should thus be viewed with caution.

A further investigation into anorexia and educational pressure was conducted by Hamburg and Herzog in 1985. These researchers asked 212 medical students to fill out a questionnaire on eating attitudes. Subjects were asked to think back to a time when they may have experienced an eating problem, and to fill in the questionnaire based on the attitudes they held during this period. From 212 subjects' responses, 19 participants were judged to meet the criteria for anorexia or bulimia nervosa. The questionnaires from these 19 women were thus analysed to establish the causes of their eating problems. The most frequently identified cause was educational pressure. Hamburg and Herzog's sample, however was taken from a population of medical students, all of whom might be expected to have experienced educational pressure at some point in their lives. Also the study was retrospective. Subjects were recruited many years after their eating problems had ceased. Such self-report designs are often highly unreliable (Sullivan, 1954).

A further retrospective study into anorexia and educational attainment was conducted by Eagles et al in 1990. This investigation analysed the case notes for 73 anorexic patients gathered between 1972 and 1979, and compared these notes to similar information gathered from 88 patients with other psychiatric diagnoses. The authors found that 79% of the anorexics had one 'O' level or better, compared to only 56% of the non-anorexic patients. Again, Eagles et al's methodology should be closely evaluated before these findings are accepted. The cut off point of one or more 'O' levels is quite arbitrary and may have helped to distort the overall impression of the educational difference between the two groups. Also the anorexic sample appear to have been younger than the non-anorexics and may therefore have had access to educational opportunities denied to the latter group.

The anorexic's place of residence

In addition to research investigating social class and education, socio-culturalists have also undertaken some limited research into the anorexic's place of residence. Although the research in this area is somewhat sparse, the conclusions appear to be that the anorexic will probably be a city dweller (Nadoka et al, 1996, Azuma and Henmi, 1982) and will almost certainly come from an 'industrial' society (Carlos, 1972, Neki, 1973). In Japan in 1996, a total of 97 eating disordered referrals were studied by Nadoka et al. The majority were from 'medium sized cities', leading the researchers to conclude that eating disorders 'are influenced by urbanization' (Nadoka et al, 1996:305). As with the investigations examining class and educational background however, Nadoka et al's methodology may have been flawed. Their 'urban' category, for example comprised cities with between 60,000 and 250,00 inhabitants. The fact that many anorexics lived in such places is hardly surprising given the all-encompassing nature of this category.

The Anorexic Stereotype – Truth or Artefact?

It is important to assess whether the anorexic stereotype is truth or artefact. The issue of whether there is any substance to the claim that anorexics are young, middle class, urban, achievers must be addressed. The physician's impression of who develops the disorder may indeed have been influenced by flawed research. If this is the case then 'working class' anorexia may always have been present but may have been missed by clinicians. An alternative explanation however is possible. Such research may initially have been accurate but may have become outdated due to the spread of anorexia more widely through society. It is noticeable that studies which support the stereotype (Morgan and Russell, 1975, Crisp et al. 1976, Szmukler et al, 1986) were conducted some years ago, while studies which have produce opposite results are more recent. Given the methodological deficiencies of many of the 'pro-stereotype' studies however, it is difficult to judge whether any confidence can be placed in their results. Maybe older, rural, working class anorexics with few educational qualifications have always been present, but have been missed. Alternatively, the characteristics which pre-dispose women towards anorexia may have proliferated throughout society, and indeed throughout the globe. A discussion of the spread of anorexia, with particular reference to globalisation, is now offered.

Globalisation of Factors leading to Anorexia Nervosa

Several authors have argued that the social conditions which give rise to anorexia have begun to permeate societies outside of the urbanised, affluent west (Dolan et al, 1990, Rathner and Messner, 1993). This globalisation of factors which lead to anorexia has been especially noted by Lee (1995, 1996, 1997). In non-western societies, Lee explains, a similar evolution of the social conditions which have historically given rise to anorexia in the west may now be taking place. Lee therefore concludes that anorexia must be studied using an 'historicised' (1995:31) approach. Anorexia will increase, Lee explains (1997:501) as a result of an 'orchestration of bio-social factors associated with industrialised capitalism'. These include an increase in consumerism (including the commodification of food) and a rise in body centred adverts. Anorexia should therefore be viewed as being 'grounded in the transnational nature of modernity' (1996:21) with the better mass communications to which modernity gives rise. The power of the media to universalise public preoccupations may nowadays have rendered many societies susceptible to anorexia.

Socio-culturalists have therefore identified important trends in relation to the global spread of anorexia. They have also investigated key issues such as class and education, and have produced important findings that provide a basis for debate. However, the methodology used by some socio-culturalists may be identified as problematic and this represents a limitation to the socio-cultural approach. Some further limitations to socio-culturalism are discussed below.

Limitations of the Socio-Culturalist Approach

Socio-culturalists have conducted a wealth of research into social dimensions of anorexia. They have attempted to identify factors which have influenced the illness but have failed to conduct a theoretical assessment of the process through which these factors have developed. Equally, the socio-culturalist approach is unable to theorise the manner in which social influences are exerted. It is not surprising therefore that Bordo, a sociologist, asserts,

> until very recently [...] the most that one could expect in the way of social or cultural analyses [of anorexia] with very few exceptions was the unavoidable recognition that anorexia related to the increasing emphasis that fashion has placed on slenderness over the last fifteen years. (1988:89)

This encapsulates the limitations of the socio-cultural approach. Socio-culturalists offer a highly simplistic model of society's influence on anorexia. They restrict this model to the simple assertion that certain agencies, (such as media and peer group) have an effect on the development of anorexia. These agencies act in concert with the demographic positioning of the anorexic as a young, urban, middle class achiever which in turn creates the conditions which can give rise to the illness. Socio-culturalists, as we have seen, identify the importance of cultural institutions, such as the media, the family and the peer group (Toro et al, 1994) in inculcating attitudes to slimming among young women. The influence such agencies exert is seen as operating in one direction only, rendering the sufferer as a passive vehicle in this model. Thin images are presented as the ideal, and these are internalised by the viewer (Garner and Garfinkel, 1980, Toro et al, 1988). More 'indirect' influences such as social class are likewise viewed as uni-directional (Gard and Freeman, 1996). The parent's status as middle class, for example, is theorised as a contributory factor to the disorder by creating high expectations from high achieving parents for their children. This leads the child to seek re-assurance in their self selected anorexia.

Clearly then, socio-culturalism contains serious limitations. In presenting its data, it fails to theorise the social dynamics through which causative agencies have developed. Even where social institutions such as the family are identified as the 'cause' of the disorder, psychiatrists tend to focus on the individual characteristics of family members, and make little reference to wider gender, social or power issues. (Even in their brief but interesting discussions of globalisation, psychiatrists tend to limit their accounts to a description of the spread of 'western' values , but fail to theorise the mechanisms by which this spread occurs). Equally, the precise causal processes which operate in anorexogenic families are never fully evaluated, and evidence to support their existence is largely anecdotal.

In traditional psychiatric discourse an analysis of the importance of society and gender is therefore absent. By ignoring gender politics psychiatry has tended to reinforce mysogynistic myths about the innate pathology of the female body. It has been left to feminist psychiatrists to develop a theory which incorporates an assessment of the importance of gender. In theorising anorexia as a disorder overwhelmingly manifested by women, feminist psychiatrists have offered invaluable insights into the causes of eating disorder. Their contribution to the anorexia debate will now be discussed.

Psychiatric Feminism

Some psychotherapists are also feminists (e.g. Orbach, 1993, Lawrence, 1995, Sesan, 1994, Fallon et al, 1994, Raymond et al, 1994, Katzman, 1993). These feminists have attempted to incorporate an analysis of patriarchy and the social role of gender, into their approach. Essentially feminism tells us that the cultural role to which women are taught to aspire is itself problematic. Anorexic behaviour is understood as violent social protest against this problematic social role. The dysfunction, however, does not reside in the psychology of the individual patient, but resides rather in the culture to which that patient belongs.

Psychiatric feminism is the approach adopted by Orbach (1993), Lawrence (1995), Sesan (1994), Katzman, (1993), Fallon et al (1994), and Raymond et al (1994).[4] These researchers theorise anorexia by locating it in a wider analysis of patriarchy. Only by addressing the wider constraints of women's lives, they suggest, can we truly address the cause of the disorder. Orbach, for example, asserts that the anorexic should be viewed as a hunger striker, a political figure engaged in protest against the injustices of patriarchal society. The anorexic's refusal to eat, in Orbach and Lawrence's view, is due less to childish recalcitrance than to the imperative of lodging a serious protest against adult femininity. In a society that objectifies women, all females are pressurised to subordinate their nutritional needs to the requirement to be thin. Lawrence (1995) therefore suggests that anor-

4 In addition, researchers such as Irigaray (1985) and Kristeva (2001) have developed a school of *psychoanalytic* feminism, based on a feminist re-working of Freudian and Lacanian psychoanalysis. Few of these authors however have concerned themselves specifically with the study of anorexia nervosa, and for this reason, I have chosen to omit them from this analysis. The chief concern of psychoanalytic feminists, (as befits a Freudian approach), appears to be the development of a detailed theory of identity construction in early infancy and the application of this theory in the therapeutic setting. The current study however, has a somewhat different focus, (that of theorising the construction of 'anorexic knowledge'). As a result, a discussion of psychoanalytic feminism will not be offered in this book.

exia should be understood as an extension of the problematic relationship all women have with food.

Limitations of Psychiatric Feminism

Psychiatric feminism has addressed some of the deficiencies of existing psychiatric theory. With the exception of adding a feminist dimension, however, such an approach is largely based on the psychiatric model. Both Orbach and Lawrence acknowledge the role of patriarchy in limiting the repertoire of emotions which women are allowed to express (Lawrence, 1995) and in commodifying women's bodies and creating body insecurity (Orbach, 1993). At the same time, however, they identify the family, and indeed the mother, as the one of the principle sources of the patient's pathology. Although Lawrence (1995), asserts that 'blaming families is probably the least helpful stand that a therapist can take' (1995:57), she nevertheless goes on to say that she has never met 'an anorexic who had a 'straightforward' relationship with her mother' (1995:67).

Even during their children's infancy, Lawrence suggests, anorexogenic mothers dysfunctionally anticipate their children's feeding needs. They feed by the clock rather than on demand, and such oversolicitous practices contribute to anorexia (Lawrence, 1995:63). Similarly Orbach (1993), has described the pathogenic 'failure' of the mother to instil a strong sense of self in her infant. Orbach (1993) suggests that anorexic mothers fail to cuddle their daughters sufficiently, subconsciously conveying that the daughter's role in life will be to meet the needs of others rather than her own. Lawrence (1995) further suggests that anorexia may be caused by guilt in the mind of the daughter derived from the mother's limited social role which the daughter is unwilling to take on. Such guilt is unlikely to manifest itself as anorexia in all women, as it only one of a number of contributing factors which combine to produce the disorder. This reproduction of the model of the anorexogenic mother is a key weakness in psychiatric feminism.

Notwithstanding the insights of psychiatric feminism this approach contains limitations. Like the 'sociological' feminism described in Chapter 2, it tends to rarefy the physical experience of anorexic women by theorising their illness in terms of an abstract political struggle. As such, anorexia is seen more as a metaphor for society than as a painful physical illness experienced by individual women. To its credit, however, psychiatric feminism also attends to some of the sufferer's individual experience (such as her relationship with her family, her struggle for control, etc.). For this reason however, psychiatric feminists (Orbach, 1993, Lawrence, 1995) are prone to reproducing the deficiencies of the psychiatric model, particularly in relation to identifying mothers as the 'cause' of the disorder. Regardless of its shortcomings however, feminism, both sociological and psychiatric, remains one of the most clearly articulated and soundly theorised expositions of anorexic aetiology.

In placing women's oppression at the centre of its analysis, feminism presents a challenge to existing psychiatric orthodoxy. Feminists however, are not the only people to have critiqued 'mainstream' psychiatry Other critics of the 'anorexic stereotype' have emerged from within psychiatry itself. Lee (1996), in particular has developed a highly articulate and compassionate critique of existing approaches, and a summary of his contribution, and the contribution of other psychiatrists in challenging the stereotype, will now be presented.

Psychiatry's challenge to the anorexic stereotype

Fat phobia

Notwithstanding the prominence of the anorexic stereotype, several psychiatrists have questioned some of its key tenets. Lee (1996) in particular has questioned the functionality of 'fat phobia' as a diagnostic criteria. Such 'fat phobia' (APA, 1980, 1994) locates the causes of anorexia in bodily pre-occupations with appearance. So well established is this idea that 'fear of fatness' is one of the most rigid and persistent bio-clinical criteria for diagnosing the illness. The symptom relates not only to a presumed terror of weight gain, but also to the cosmetic strategy of dieting to address this fear. The anorexic is thus presented as a vain, appearance obsessed, youngster whose dieting has simply 'got out of control'. Such a portrayal may mask the deeper, very troubling psychological causes that have led to the disorder.

In Lee's (1996) view, cosmetic concerns surrounding weight gain may be only secondary to deeper underlying causes. Fear of fatness, Lee argues may be a highly 'western' symptom. For non-western, oriental women, (many of whom report other reasons for dieting, such as 'fear of being too greedy'), fat phobia may be unimportant. Szekley (1989) also discovered that fat loathing, and the search for thinness, though highly specific activities, did not always derive from the same motivation. Different women had different reasons for wanting to be thin, and their life circumstances and the meaning dieting held for them were often very varied.

By constructing anorexia as a disorder which is concerned with cosmetic appearance, existing models 'miss the broader contexts and varied meanings of food refusal' (Katzman and Lee, 1997:385). Thus 'the concerns of the typical patient are sorted along bodily dimensions while other concerns are potentially erased' (Katzman and Lee, 1997:390). Lee is a psychiatrist, and it is important to emphasise that the first criticisms of fat phobia originated among psychiatrists themselves. In the mind of many clinicians, however, (APA, 1980, 1994), fear of fatness remains one of the key causes of anorexia.

Class

As well as fat phobia, other aspects of the 'anorexic stereotype', especially in relation to class have also been challenged from within the clinical community, particularly by Gard and Freeman in 1996. It is important to be clear in this book that the contention that class and anorexia are unlinked, originated with these clinicians.

Gard and Freeman performed a review of journal articles from the 1970s to the 1990s. While early articles, Gard and Freeman explain, proposed a relationship between anorexia and social class, papers from the mid 1980s showed no such correlation. Gard and Freeman thus concluded that the social class bias in earlier studies may simply have reflected a greater 'willingness' on the part of middle class families, 'to seek psychiatric help' (1996:3). 'It is interesting' the authors suggest, 'how a clinical myth builds up evidence to support the myth' (1996:6). Despite this, the authors concluded that the middle class 'stereotype remains firmly entrenched', a conclusion supported by Rogers et al in 1997. In a study of 1757 adolescents, however, Rogers et al observed that while middle class girls dieted more often than working class girls, there was no class difference in reported incidence of eating disorders.

The absence of any class bias in the area of anorexia was also noted by Whitaker et al in 1989. Whitaker et al conducted a study of 5596 students who were given the Eating Symptoms Inventory and the Eating Attitudes Test (Garner and Garfinkel, 1979). Subjects were also asked whether they had dieted in the previous 12 months. While girls from social classes 1 and II were more likely to have been on a diet, high EAT and ESI scores were unrelated to social class, leading the authors to conclude that class and anorexia were not linked.

Clearly therefore the current study is not the first to challenge the bio-medical stereotype of anorexia nervosa. What the current study does do however is to evaluate several different aspects of the stereotype – e.g. fat phobia, class, and educational level, in the same sample. In so doing it presents a far more rigorous challenge to studies which selectively examine limited aspects of the bio-medical model. Also, unlike previous studies, the current investigation examines the transmission, (as well as the existence), of the clinical stereotype, and as such represents an advance over previous research. Nevertheless, existing studies, (e.g. Lee, 1991, Gard and Freeman, 1996, Whitaker et al, 1989) as this section has demonstrated, constitute an established challenge to the anorexic stereotype – a challenge that has originated from within psychiatry itself. The emergence of such dissent indicates that the discipline of psychiatry is dynamic rather than static. The models described so far in this chapter have been presented largely in a static form, with only passing reference to the manner in which these models have changed over time. To illustrate the process by which psychiatric thought can alter, I will now appraise the changing content of some selected psychiatric texts. The texts I have chosen are the key books recommended to medical students studying psychiatry (Kaplan and Sadock, 1995, Gelder et al, 2004, Russell, 2000, APA, 1994). An appraisal of these texts will now be offered.

Texts recommended to medical students over the past 25 years

The suggestion that medical knowledge is dynamic and subject to change, was made in Chapter 1. Mizrachi (2002) was one of several authors cited in relation to this issue. Mizrachi described the way in which the medical conceptualisation of anorexia between 1939–1979 had altered, with physical manifestations (such as weight loss) becoming privileged over time (see Chapter 1). Mizrachi's analysis goes up to 1979, but post 1979 developments may be traced by examining material in psychiatric textbooks published since the early 1980s (APA, 1980, APA, 1994, Gelder et al, 2004, 1983, Gelder et al, 2000, Russell, 2000, Kaplan and Sadock, 1995, 1985, 1967). In conducting this analysis, I have particularly focussed on textbooks used in medical schools during this period.

There are at present 34 medical schools in the UK (Council of Heads of Medical Schools Website, 2005: http://www.chms.ac.uk). I selected 17 schools from this list and accessed the websites of these schools. For 9 of these schools I was able to access on-line information for modules on the 'B.Sc. Medical Studies'[5] programmes. Each programme contained either a level 2 or level 3 introductory psychiatry module. I obtained reading lists for these modules for each of the 9 institutions. For the remaining 8 schools, I emailed departmental secretaries, and explained I was conducting research into 'how psychiatrists describe anorexia'. Two secretaries sent me reading lists for their level 3 psychiatry modules.

To gather longitudinal data, I phoned 7 module leaders, (using the on-line contact numbers for their schools). I asked these tutors how long they had been in post and how long specific texts had been recommended. Two module leaders had taught psychiatry for 17 years and 24 years respectively. During this time, they explained, key reference texts had not altered significantly. I obtained further longitudinal data by phoning the libraries and bookshops of 10 schools. At three universities information was provided from library staff of many years standing. They explained that the texts they stocked had remained consistent during this period.

This search indicated that one manual had been consistently used at least since the early eighties. This, of course, was the *Diagnostic and Statistical Manual* (APA, 1968, APA, 1980, APA, 1994) first published in 1968. This had featured as a 'permanent' fixture on reading lists, as it forms the schematic basis by which medical diagnoses are made. In an era of evidence based medicine (Sackett et al, 1997), students are encouraged more and more strenuously to consult such manuals as sources of best practice and, while this material has always being important, it may now be referred to even more widely than previously.

5 Medical students complete this three-year programme prior to completing their MD qualification.

The DSM is periodically updated and criteria for making its diagnoses are revised. It is currently in its fourth edition (DSM-IV), which contains a highly medicalised definition of anorexia, centring on fat phobia, weight loss, and physical symptoms such as the loss of the menses (see page 25). Earlier editions of the DSM make reference to anorexia as a single diagnosis. In later versions, however, a subtype of anorexia 'bulimarexia', is specified. This describes the condition whereby weight loss is maintained through self-induced vomiting, rather than food restriction. Such a definition is consistent with the DSM's emphasis on somatic symptoms of anorexia.

As well as the DSM, three textbooks were consistently recommended from the early 1980s onwards. Two of these textbooks were Oxford publications – *The Shorter Oxford Textbook of Psychiatry* (Gelder et al, 2004, first published in 1983) and *The New Oxford Textbook of Psychiatry* (Gelder et al, 2000, (eds.), chapter on 'Eating Disorders' by Russell, 2000). An American textbook, (Kaplan and Sadock, 1995, first printed in 1967), also appeared. This explained that prevailing psychological approaches (e.g. psychoanalysis in 30s 40s and 50s) may influence the way anorexia is explained at a given social moment. This was supported by the Oxford Textbook, which suggested that the form and content of anorexia has changed over time.

Each book presented a bio-medical model of anorexia based on DSM criteria, (though later editions stressed multi-causal explanations). In such editions socio-cultural issues featured more fully alongside the medical model. Acknowledging societal influences, Russell stresses the 'cult of thinness' as central to inducing 'weight phobia' suggesting 'modern societal pressures have determined the patient's [...] food avoidance' (2000:837). In providing this explanation however, no reference is made to feminist thought, except in very recent editions of the American text.

The model of the anorexic as young, female, western and middle class is also presented (though authors had little to say about the anorexic's level of education). The British textbooks clearly state that anorexia is a disorder of the middle class. 'The condition is more common', suggest Gelder et al, 'in the upper than the lower social classes' (2004:447). Later editions of the American textbook disagree however. Class and anorexia, Kaplan et al suggest, are no longer linked, and anorexics may come from any social class. This difference in opinion reflects the changing nature of anorexic knowledge, and gives further support to the challenge to the anorexic stereotype from within psychiatry (see pages 102–4). It also indicates one of the few areas in which accounts differed in the American and British textbooks. Apart from this difference, the discussion of anorexia was very similar in all publications, where family systems theory (see page 83) and obsessional personality disorder, were used to theorise the disorder. In the newer editions, however, the term 'obsessional' was used much more frequently, while 'fear of maturity' was 'down-played'.

This appraisal of clinical textbooks suggests that clinical interpretations of anorexia fluctuate over time. A relatively consistent feature of such explanations however is their focus on physiological issues. This was most apparent in the 'Shorter Oxford' where physiological factors (low blood pressure, cold sensitivity and the loss of the menarche) were 'flagged up' at the outset. In this shortened account, it would appear that key elements of the anorexic stereotype (fat phobia, youth and high social class) were more to the fore. While supporting a multi-factorial explanation, all the medical textbooks presented chapters in which the clinical model clearly predominated.

Conclusion

This chapter has described psychiatric approaches to the study of anorexia nervosa. It has identified that psychiatrists have applied a 'family systems' (Minuchin et al, 1978) model to the analysis of the illness. This approach has analysed anorexia in terms of relational dynamics in the sufferer's family of origin. Such families are identified as enmeshed, inward looking and uncommunicative. Social status is prioritised in such families and is valued over genuine demonstrations of love and support.

Psychiatry has also developed a highly distinct template for 'typical' manifestations of anorexia nervosa. This template comprises symptoms such as fear of maturity, fat phobia, control and perfectionism. This book will argue that this template constitutes a stereotype of the anorexic's cognitive symptoms. 'Socio-cultural' psychiatrists have also produced a stereotype. This consists of the 'typical' social group from which the sufferer comes. This group is identified as young, urban, middle class, and high achieving (Morgan and Russell, 1975, Crisp et al 1976, Nadoka et al, 1996, Hamburg and Herzog, 1985). More recent studies however have suggested that anorexics come from a wide range of socio-economic groups and places of residence, and have a variety of educational qualifications (Gard and Freeman, 1996, Rathner and Messner, 1993). Nevertheless, the stereotype of the bright, affluent, urban anorexic persists in spite of growing evidence of its inaccuracy.

Existing psychiatric approaches therefore have significant limitations. Some of these limitations have been addressed by feminists (Orbach, 1993, Lawrence, 1995). These feminist psychiatrists have integrated an analysis of patriarchy and gender into patient therapy. They have identified the importance of women's disempowerment in the development of anorexia, and have thus explained that the pathology which gives rise to anorexia can be located in society rather than in the psychology of the individual. Feminism is not the only source of opposition to the stereotype, however. A further challenge has been brought by psychiatrists themselves. Such a challenge emphasises that different women have different reasons for dieting, and that these women come from a variety of social classes. An appraisal of psychiatric textbooks suggests that psychiatric knowledge changes over time and that more psychiatrists now acknowledge 'working class' anorexia. Social class, together with age, education and place of residence, are important issues in any discussion of anorexia. The results gathered in the current study for these items are presented in the next chapter.

Chapter 5
The Demographic Profile of the Patient Sample

Introduction

In the last chapter I discussed the key elements of the psychiatric model of anorexia. One of these elements concerned the demographic profile typically attributed to the anorexic patient. This chapter aims to dismantle some of the myths surrounding the demographic stereotype. Previous research (Gard and Freeman, 1996, Lee, 1996) has addressed aspects of the stereotype, for example those that relate to social class. No study prior to this one, however, has addressed several dimensions of the stereotype in the same sample. By presenting data on age, class, education and place of residence from 104 anorexics, this chapter aims to demonstrate that anorexics are from both the middle and working classes, are both high and low achievers, are of various ages, and have grown up in all kinds of geographical areas.

Between 1985 and 1990, a study of eating disorder was conducted in a district general hospital (Palmer et al, 1990). I was part of the team that conducted this investigation. The study collected data on age, social class, education and place of residence from 80 anorexic and 78 bulimic patients. All patients were consecutive referrals to the Eating Disorders Unit, and all had met DSM-III criteria (APA, 1980) for anorexia or bulimia nervosa. Data on age and class from the combined sample of bulimic and anorexic patients was published in 1990 (Palmer et al), but similar data for the sample of anorexic patients only have not previously been published. Also, no data have hitherto been published on education and place of residence for either the anorexic or the bulimic group.

The results presented in this book are compiled from the anorexic group only. As discussed in Chapter 3, these have been combined with data from an additional sample of 24 (DSM-IV, APA, 1994) anorexics, recruited from the same unit between 1997 and 2001. Data from a total of 104 anorexic patients are therefore presented in this chapter. These data are compared to Census data, (OPCS, 1997) on class and residence, and Department of Education data on educational attainment (1996, 2000).

In the following section results are presented describing the sex, age, class, education and place of residence of the anorexic sample. For some of these variables, small proportions of cases are missing. These represent those women who chose not to supply information for these items on the questionnaire. These items were coded as missing, and were removed from the frequency and percentage columns (and from the total calculations) in the following tables. Statistical calculations are based on real values only.

Anorexia and Sex

All but three of the anorexic participants (97%) were female. What is interesting about this finding is that it demonstrates that one element of the anorexic stereotype is accurate. Anorexics are almost always women. It is therefore appropriate to ask what is it about being a woman that increases the risk of contracting the disorder. Feminists (Chernin, 1986, MacSween, 1993) have suggested that anorexia results from the contradictory expectations conveyed to women in patriarchal society. As MacSween (1993), explains women are nominally encouraged to achieve in public life, but are in practice excluded from a masculine dominated culture. As a result of their subsequent disempowerment, women turn to food as an area over which they can exert control.

Women are also conditioned to view their bodies in negative terms. Women's bodies are constructed as open, passive and complementary to the male (MacSween, 1993). The male body is constructed as the norm against which the female body is constructed as other. The resulting objectification of women's bodies can lead to body insecurity (Orbach, 1993), which can create the conditions in which anorexia can thrive.

While very few of the anorexic patients were male, the fact of there being any requires some comment. Without question, male sufferers of anorexia have been largely ignored in the literature (Cantrell and Ellis, 1991). This is beginning to change (Frasciello and Willard, 1995), but nevertheless, the overwhelming body of anorexic research has centred on female sufferers. This has lead some commentators to erroneously describe anorexia as uniquely feminine (Boskind-White and White, 1986). It is often suggested that socio cultural pressures put women more at risk from developing the disorder because of society's emphasis on thinness as a major element of feminine identity. Clinical evidence however (Frasciello and Willard, 1995, Robinson and Holden, 1986, Herzog et al, 1984) suggests that anorexia does occur in men and that its course, prognosis and symptom profile is similar for males and females.

There is a tendency in the literature to feminise the role identity of male sufferers. The sexual orientation (Robinson and Holden, 1986) of male sufferers is frequently discussed (unlike that of females), and patients are often described as homosexual or as having limited sexual experience (Robinson and Holden, 1986). Cantrell and Ellis however (1991), have discussed anorexia in relation to the social role evolution of males and females. As women become more emancipated, the current evolutionary point of the masculine gender role also changes, and men may become more objectified. As men see their bodies increasingly attached to adverts for Diet Coke and other consumables, they too may fall prey to anorexia and bulimia nervosa.

Anorexia and Age

Age is frequently identified as a distinguishing characteristic in relation to anorexia nervosa (Bruch, 1978, Rastam et al, 1989). Anorexia is almost universally identified as a young woman's disorder and most anorexics are believed to come from the 15–19 age group (Lucas et al, 1988). It is generally considered that even women who experience the disorder in adulthood will have first contracted anorexia when in their teens. The age of onset for anorexic symptoms, is therefore usually considered to be during puberty or early adulthood. One paper, however (Wills and Olivieri, 1988) suggests that women may experience the disorder throughout the course of their adult lives. They may become anorexic in their forties and fifties, and even occasionally into their 'old age'. In the current study, age distribution was as follows:

Table 5.1: Age Distribution – The Anorexic Sample

	Frequency	Percent
15 to 19	30	29.7
20 to 29	51	50.5
30 to 39	13	12.8
40 to 49	4	4.0
Over 50	3	3.0
Total	101	100

(Missing 3)

The average age of the anorexic sample was 24.9 (sd: 8.7, range 15 to 59). The largest age group was the 20–29 age group (50.5%). Many of the anorexic sample (29.7%) were under 20, supporting the findings of previous studies, (Bruch, 1978, Hindler et al, 1994) which suggest that anorexia is predominantly a disease of young women. There were however, also a number of older (> 30 years) women (19.9% of the anorexic sample) which demonstrates that anorexia is not purely confined to the young. This calls into question the clinical stereotype of anorexics as almost universally a young women's disorder.

Anorexia and Social Class

Significant controversy continues to surround debates about anorexia and social class. In the 1970s and 1980s, a key feature of the stereotype anorexic was that she would be from one of the higher socio-economic groups (Crisp et al, 1976, Szmukler et al, 1986). Such an individual would be subject to all of the behavioural pressures characteristic of the middle class. These include the pressure to 'keep up appearances', to achieve, and to comply with family expectations without complaint (Bruch, 1978). Such pressures, it is argued, create an environment in which anorexia may develop.

In the current study, class was allocated using the Registrar General's (OPCS, 1980) classification of occupations. This system was used as the majority of study data were gathered in the 1980s and the early 1990s. According to the Registrar General's classification, class is organised in a descending scale, with the most privileged and well paid (for example doctors and lawyers) occupying social class 1, and the least privileged (road sweepers, cleaners) occupying social class 5. The registrar general's classification has been identified as problematic in recent years, particularly in relation to women (Townsend and Davidson, 1992:312, Acheson, 1998:31), who often continue to be classified in relation to their husbands. In addition, there are wider problems with this scheme as it is 'based on a male occupational structure' (Annandale, 1998:149). When transposing female employment onto the scheme, women tend to become clustered into a limited range of occupational classes (e.g.'class 3 non-manual [...] and to a lesser extent as class 2', Annandale, 1998:149). In the current study, adult women were classified according to their own occupation, but the wider problems with the OPCS classifications remain and the following social class data should be read in this light.

In addition to supplying information on their own occupation, participants were also asked to state the occupation of their parents. Many of the anorexic subjects were young people, and had developed their illness while still living at home. It was felt that in these cases parental occupation might be used as a guide to the subject's social class of origin. For younger subjects (< 18 years) therefore, both mother's and father's occupation were recorded, and social class was derived from the higher of the two occupations. These social class data were then compared to census data for the geographical area from which referrals to the unit were made (OPCS, 1997). Using this scheme the social class distribution of the anorexic and census group was as follows:

Table 5.2: Social Class – The Anorexic Sample and National Census Data		
The Anorexic Sample		
	Frequency	Percent
Social Class 1	4	4.0
Social Class 2	23	23.0
Social Class 3 Non-manual	21	21.0
Social Class 3 Manual	12	12.0
Social Class 4	8	8.0
Social Class 5	13	13.0
Other	19	19.0
Total	100	100
(Missing 4)		
National Census Data (1991)*		
	Frequency: Number of families**	Percent
Social Class 1	77200	6.0
Social Class 2	302249	23.0
Social Class 3 Non-manual	121541	9.0
Social Class 3 Manual	264227	20.0
Social Class 4	35844	3.0
Social Class 5	98354	8.0
Other	397383	31.0
Total	1296798	100

Source: Office of Population Censuses and Surveys (1993), *1991 Census report for Great Britain*, London: HMSO, p.333.

*Ten per cent sample recoded to Registrar General's 1980 categories (classified according to occupation of head of household)

**A proportion of these families may have had a member with anorexia. Hoek (1991) estimates the incidence rate for anorexia as 6.3 per 100,000.

Table 5.2 (cont.): Social Class* – The Anorexic Sample and National Census Data		
Anorexics by General Population:		
	Anorexics (%)	General Population (1991 Census) (%)
Middle Class	48%	38%
Working Class	52%	62%
Total	100%	100%

* (Social Class 1, 2 and 3-Non Manual) recoded into 'Middle class'
(Social Class 3-Manual, 4, 5 and Other) recoded into 'Working class'
$\chi2 = 2.040$ df (1) (Not significant)

A clear trend is in evidence here. For social classes 1 and 2, there appears to be no difference between the anorexic sample and 'normal' people (as measured by the census). Social classes 1 and 2 account for 27% of the anorexic sample, and 29% of the census data. The key contention advanced by many psychiatrists therefore, that anorexia is predominantly a disorder experienced by women from the higher socio economic groups, would appear not to be supported by data in this study.

For social classes 3 also the overall figures (33% of anorexics, 29% of census data) are similar for the anorexics and census data. However a much higher proportion of anorexics (21%) appear in social class 3 non-manual, compared to the census (9%). Conversely a higher proportion of social class 3 manual appear in the census data (20%) when compared to the anorexics (12%).

This may be because census data is derived from the occupation of 'heads of households', most of which are recorded as men. As Annandale, (1998), explains a much higher proportion of social class 3 non-manual are female, while social class 3 manual is predominantly male.

Some sociologists have suggested that members of social class 3 non-manual are middle, rather than working class. The clean, safe conditions of work, and the paid holidays which many clerks, tele-salespeople, shop workers and hotel receptionists, etc. enjoy, are sometimes cited as evidence of the higher socio-economic status of these groups. Nevertheless, these (predominantly female) sectors contain some of the most ‘low level’ jobs in society (Crompton, 1998:150). Such sectors are therefore difficult to categorise, and may even be ‘extended’ working, rather than middle, class (Wright, 1997:244). Also, female employment, when measured by the OPCS, tends to become clustered in the 3 non-manual category (see page 113). Consequently, in terms of class, these women may have more in common with their working class ‘male counterparts’ (in social class 3 manual), than with higher socio-economic groups.

I support this latter argument and therefore contend that anorexic patients come from all socio-economic groups. The class distribution among my anorexic subjects was not significantly different to that observed among census data. These results suggest that both working class and middle class women may and do develop anorexia.

Anorexia and Education

Anorexic subjects were asked to state their highest educational qualification. These data were then compared to Department of Education data (DoE, 2000) on national educational attainment. Surprisingly, the anorexic sample appeared to have achieved at lower level than women generally (with 22% of women recorded by the DoE having a university degree compared to 10% of anorexics – see Table 5.3).

This may be because many anorexics (n=80) were recruited to the study some years before the DoE data was recorded, during which time access to higher education has improved (see Table 5.5). However, anorexics were largely young women (table 5.1) and potentially had better access to higher education than the ‘average aged’ women in the DoE figures. Nevertheless, the comparatively older women in the DoE survey were higher educational achievers. Access to higher education has significantly improved in the last 15 years (table 5.5), but regardless of year of comparison, the figures for degree standard education are higher in the general employed workforce (14 % in 1985, and 20% in 1995) than for the anorexics in the current study (10.2%). This indicates that anorexics are no more likely than the general population to excel in the educational sphere.

At the time of their interview, however some anorexics were so young they might not have been old enough to have finished university, and this may also have distorted the figures. Even when this is accounted for however, the anorexic sample appeared to be achieving less well than their peers. It is not surprising that when one experiences a serious psychiatric illness one's education should suffer. Lengthy stays in a psychiatric hospital, preceded by the trauma leading to admission might reasonably be expected to materially affect educational development. What is surprising however is the relatively modest educational attainment observed in this study among a group of women who are often identified as high achievers (Eagles et al, 1990, Bruch, 1978).

Anorexia and Place of Residence

In existing research, a stereotypical approach may also be evident with regard to the anorexic's place of residence. Although research into this issue is limited, there appears to be a stereotype of the anorexic as a city dweller (Nadoka et al, 1996, Azuma and Henmi, 1982) from an 'industrialised' country (Carlos, 1972, Neki, 1973, German, 1972). Such a suggestion is consistent with the sophisticated urban lifestyle with its emphasis on image and bodywork that some researchers believe gives rise to anorexia. Once again however, as with social class, previous research has gathered inconclusive results in relation to this issue. Azuma and Henmi in 1982 found that anorexia nervosa was four times more common in a big city (Kyoto), than in the surrounding rural area, while Nadoka et al (1996) also found that the

Table 5.3: Educational Attainment – The Anorexic Sample and Department of Education Data		
The Anorexic Sample		
	Frequency	Percent
Degree and above	10	10.2
'A' Level	19	19.2
GCSE/GCE 'O' Level	28	28.3
Other	27	27.2
None	15	15.1
Total	99	100
(Missing 5)		
Department of Education Data 2000		
Females of Working Age* (000s)		
	Frequency	Percent
Degree and above	3805	22.0
'A' Level	2420	14.0
GCSE/GCE 'O' Level	3805	22.0
Other	3977	23.0
None	3285	19.0
Total	17,292	100

*A proportion of these women may have had anorexia. Hoek (1991) estimates the incidence rate for anorexia as 6.3 per 100,000.
Source: Education and Training statistics for the United Kingdom: 2000, Department for Education and Employment, London:HMSO. p.85

Table 5.4: Education: Anorexics by General Population		
	Anorexics (%)	General Population (%) (Dept of Education Data 2000)
'A' Level or above	29.4	36
Below 'A' Level	70.6	64
Total	100	100

$\chi2$ = 1.117 df (1) (Not significant)
Source: Education and Training statistics for the United Kingdom: 2000, Department for Education and Employment, London:HMSO. p.85

Table 5.5: Improvements in Educational Qualifications in the General Population 1985–1995											
	1985	1986	1987	1988	1989	1990	1991	1992	1993	1994	1995
Degree or equivalent *											
East Midlands	14	14	13	14	13	15	16	17	19	21	20
England	16	16	16	16	16	17	17	20	22	23	23
Two 'A' Levels or equivalent *											
East Midlands	25	24	23	25	25	27	29	29	34	37	37
England	27	27	27	27	28	29	30	33	38	40	40
Five GCSE or equiva-lent**											
East Midlands	39	40	43	45	47	53	50	57	59	62	70
England	45	44	46	47	50	51	53	58	61	64	64

* percentage of employed workforce
** percentage of 19–21 year olds
Source: Education statistics for the United Kingdom: 1995, Department for Education and Employment (1996), London:HMSO. p.86–7
A proportion of these families may have had a member with anorexia. Hoek (1991) estimates the incidence rate for anorexia as 6.3 per 100,000.

majority of their sample of 97 eating disordered subjects came from medium sized cities. In other studies however the opposite trend has been noted. In 1991 for example, Hoek found that anorexia occurred with almost equal frequency in rural areas when compared to cities, while Rathner and Messner (1993) found a 'high' rate of eating disorder among 517 schoolgirls from a small Italian town.

In the current study, respondents were asked to describe the size of the town in which they grew up. The residence profile of the anorexics was then compared to residence data for the whole country from the 1991 census (table 5.6). When compared to these data, the figure for residents of large cities was much higher in the general population (32%) than in the anorexic sample (15.6%). The findings (table 5.6) also show that anorexics were more likely than census subjects to come from small towns and rural areas. These data support the findings of Hoek (1991) and Rathner and Messner (1993) and cast doubt on the notion of the stereotype anorexic as an urbanised city dweller.

A Discussion of the Demographic Findings from the Current Study

According to the above findings, only two elements of the anorexic stereotype are supported. Anorexics are almost universally women, and are usually, though not always, young. Other elements of the anorexic stereotype (concerning social class, education and residence) would appear to have little empirical support. The results of the current study indicate that anorexics are not overwhelmingly middle class, highly educated achievers from big cities, and this requires some comment.

Social class

This study clearly suggests that both working class and middle class women get anorexia. Yet in spite of growing evidence to the contrary (Whitaker et al, 1989, Lee, 1991, Rogers et al, 1997), the stereotype of the middle class anorexic continues to hold sway in academic and clinical environments (Gelder et al, 2004). As Gard and Freeman (1996:1) explain,

> the prevailing wisdom concerning the relationship between eating disorders and socio-economic status in both the professional and the lay person's mind is that there is an increased prevalence of eating disorders in high socio-economic status groups.

This misconception may be due to the powerful influence of clinical impression (Gard and Freeman, 1996). In the course of their clinical practice doctors normally encounter middle class anorexic patients (Hoek, 1993). Bias in the referral system (Zola, 1973, Blaxter, 1981) may mean that middle class girls are more likely to be referred to specialist services. The 'soldiering on' and 'what will be' fatalism (Zola, 1966, Taylor and Field, 1993, Graham, 1984) among the working class may result in women from lower socio-economic groups deciding not to trouble their GPs, even though they might have a serious eating disorder.

A further reason for the persistence of the middle class stereotype may be that roughly two decades ago, 'poor' girls did not get anorexia. Working class girls may have begun to contract the disorder only in the past decade or so, and as a result, cases of working class anorexia would have seldom appeared in earlier studies. Szmukler and colleagues (1986:49), for example suggest that changes have occurred

> in subjects now presenting with the illness with an increase in older patients, in those who are married or sexually experienced and with more patients coming from social backgrounds which were previously considered non conducive to the development of the illness, for example lower social class.

Szmukler et al (1986:49) explain that this may be due to the socio-cultural factors which contribute to anorexia 'spreading more widely through society'. Such a perspective would argue that the conditions which contribute to anorexia, (such as deferred gratification and valuation of thinness) have seeped down from the middle class into lower socio-economic groups. As anorexia has become increasingly glamourised (see Chapter 9), working class girls may have 'caught up' with

Table 5.6: Place of Residence when Growing up: Anorexics by the General Poplation		
The Anorexic Sample		
	N	% of total
City	15	15.7
Large town	15	15.7
Middle sized town	30	31.6
Small market town	13	13.7
Village	20	21.0
Farm	2	2.3
Total	95	100
(Missing 9)		
National Census Data (1991)*		
Size of Connurbation	Population	
	N	% of total
1,000,000 and over	13,268,952	32
500,000–999,999	3,465,888	8
200,000–499,999	5,962,431	14
100,000–199,999	3,982,156	10
50,000–99,999	4,058,351	10
20,000–49,999	3,790,146	9
10,000–19,999	2,652,687	6
5,000–9,999	2,027,109	5
2,000–4,999	2,121,493	5
Under 2,000	447,386	1
Total (population of England)	41,776,599	100

Source: OPCS (1997), 1991 Census: Key statistics for urban and rural areas, p.336.

*A proportion of these people may have had anorexia. Hock (1991) estimates the incidence rate for anorexia as 6.3 per 100,000.

Table 5.7 Place of residence:* Anorexics by General Population (1991 Census)

	Anorexics (%)	General Population (1991 Census) (%)
Large Town/ City	31.4	64
Smaller than a large town/city	68.6	36
Total	100	100

*Questionnaire categories 'Large Town/ City' were mapped onto the census categories of 'conurbations of over 99,999 people'

$\chi 2 = 21.835$ df (1) (Significant in opposite direction to that expected)

their middle class counterparts in assimilating risk factors for the disorder.

This 'trickle down' model may account for some recent cases of working class anorexia. The majority of these cases however can be differently explained. Working class women may have always been at risk from eating disorder but their distress may have been largely ignored. What is interesting about Szmukler et al's (1986) observation is that it may reflect not so much the manner in which pre-disposing factors for anorexia have spread throughout society, but rather the extent to which doctors are now more prepared to acknowledge this. It is interesting to ponder why this change in clinical focus has occurred at this point in time. This may be the result of a shift in medicine's 'organizational context' (Fisher, 2001:134) towards a more 'client-centred', 'classless' practice. As Fisher explains, 'because this organizational context developed over time and in response to particular moments in history, it is amenable to change – time has passed and we are now facing a new historical moment' (Fisher, 2001:134). If clinicians as a profession now accept the distress of lower class women and the extent to which these women are at risk from anorexia, research into 'working class' anorexia may increase. This process, by which the medical profession begins to acknowledge the suffering of lower socio-economic groups,[1] is an interesting illustration of the manner in which at-risk groups are clinically constructed.

1 See also Helman's (1987) work on heart disease.

In view of recent findings on working class anorexia, one might expect a shift in clinical focus towards a perspective which actively theorises what it is about being working class which may lead to the illness. No such interest however appears to have been generated. Researchers appear unconcerned about how the specific experiences of being working class may contribute to anorexia. Unlike psychiatry's interest in elucidating the characteristics of middle class life which give rise to the disorder, such as rigidity and high expectations, no such theoretical activity has been applied to analysing anorexia in the working class. Class-related causes of the illness among working class subjects therefore remain untheorised. But with a little analytical effort, theorising the causes of working class anorexia is a straightforward process. In response to my findings that working class women get the disorder, I want to examine in this book what it is about being working class that has led these women to develop this illness. It may be argued that the norms of working class life are as likely to contribute to anorexia as the norms of middle class life.

Anorexia for example, is frequently theorised as an attempt to restore control in circumstances where the sufferer has experienced a lack of control in other areas. Clearly, 'loss of control' is a feature of working class existence (Graham, 1984, Taylor and Field, 1993, Stacey, 1988, Blaxter, 1981). Working class girls are comparatively more likely, for example, to experience the trauma of abuse, both sexual and physical (Finkelhor, 1981, Marsh, 1994, Simoni and Ng, 2002). The loss in the victim's locus of control attendant on such experiences is well documented (Palmer et al, 1990, Fatout, 1993, O'Neil and Kerig, 2000). The response to such a trauma may well be to seek re-assurance in the rigidity of anorexia.

Similarly, the sufferer of anorexia may have experienced abuse from age-mates (see Chapter 7), and evidence suggests that anorexia is linked to being teased at school (Davis, 1995). The role of appearance in peer abuse (Crozier and Skliopidou, 2002, Olweus, 1995, Callaghan and Joseph, 1995) may render working class girls as susceptible to teasing as their middle class counterparts. The visible display of expensive, fashionable clothes (provided by middle class parents) can signal one's superiority and act as a powerful deterrent against would-be bullies. For less conspicuously 'cool' youngsters, the opposite process applies, and such girls may be easy targets.

While the study findings refute the clinical stereotype of anorexics as mainly middle class, it is important to explain that the current study is not the first investigation to problematise the stereotype of the affluent anorexic. In 1996, Gard and Freeman presented a review of research in which the social class of anorexics was recorded. Gard and Freeman indicate that studies from the mid 1980s show no relationship between anorexia and high socio-economic status. Similarly, Whitaker et al, (1989) in a large scale community survey, found that anorexia was unlinked to social class – a finding supported by Rogers et al (1997) (see Chapter 4). The suggestion that anorexics may not be predominately middle class therefore originated with these scholars and not in the current study. Unlike other studies however, the current investigation examines several dimensions of the clinical stereotype, (as well as class) in the same sample. One such dimension is education and it is to a discussion of this issue that I now turn.

Education

A similar critique to the argument made in relation to class may be made in relation to anorexia and educational attainment. The current study has found no relation between high educational achievement and being anorexic. Among clinicians however, there has been no attempt to theorise why some anorexics are comparatively low achievers, since this is not consistent with their stereotype. It has long been understood that education is linked to class (Miller, 1970, Biddle, 2001) and that class is linked to health (Platt and Thomas, 1993, Acheson, 1998). Middle class youngsters fare better in the classroom than their working class counterparts (Miller, 1970, Biddle, 2001, McCallum and Demie, 2001, Chitty, 2002) and are also more healthy (Acheson, 1998, Townsend and Davidson, 1992). Similarly, research suggests (Wadsworth, 1986) that ill health may influence one's class of attainment (and corresponding educational achievement), as well as one's class of origin. The link between both class and health on the one hand and class and education on the other, may therefore lead one to hypothesise that that health and education are also related. It is understandable that when one contracts a serious psychiatric disorder this may have an effect on educational progression. Anorexia is a chronic disorder and can prevent the sufferer from engaging in normal activities for a person her age. These activities include educational endeavour. No attempt however has been made by clinicians to theorise the negative effects of anorexia on educational development. Findings which undermine the anorexic stereotype, usually result in the conclusion that anorexia and education are not linked. No further attempt is made to theorise what these findings may mean.

City size

Findings from the current study suggest that anorexia is experienced by women from both urban and rural areas. In previous research, similar results have been presented in terms of the spread of a global urban culture through information technology and the mass media into more remote areas (Rathner and Messner, 1993). In other words, rural women may now get anorexia as a result of urbanised culture encroaching on specifically rural ways of life. A paternalistic assumption that 'down home', 'close to the soil' lifestyles are inconsistent with anorexia pervades this perspective (Azuma and Henmi, 1982). Just as there is a paternalistic suggestion that winning one's bread through daily labour, (i.e. being working class), protects against the disorder, so there may be an assumption that living off the land in a rural environment offers a similar safeguard (Azuma and Henmi, 1982). The results gathered in the current study appear to demonstrate that this may not be the case. Women from rural areas as well as those from cities are at equal risk of developing the disorder. This is in spite of the fact that such women, being geographically distant from specialist clinics, may be less likely to be referred to these services. Once again the stereotype constructed by the psychiatric research community would appear to have little basis in reality.

Conclusion – The Positivist Approach to Anorexia Nervosa

It is appropriate to ask why the anorexic stereotype persists in spite of mounting evidence of its inaccuracy. The twin explanations of referral bias and clinical impression, do not fully account for the power of the stereotype. I would argue that origins of the anorexic stereotype also lie in the epistemological approach applied to studying anorexia. Almost all studies, which have investigated eating disorder, have been conducted from a positivist perspective. At this point it is worth noting something about the current study. This study itself uses positivist methodology in order to debunk clinical constructions developed out of a positivist tradition. But the approach to establishing certainty in clinical science represents a materially more rigid framework than that adopted in this book. Several studies (for example Kutchins and Kirk, 1997) have critiqued the clinical construction of clinical diagnoses and the claims to certainty which such knowledge represents. Like the current study, these studies have also referred to findings which refute such clinical certainties, and which demonstrate that such constructions may frequently be unsupported by data. This is the established methodology used by every study which problematises positivist clinical certainty (Young, 1992, Berg and Mol, 1998, Seale et al, 2001) and thus it is the approach used in this book. My conclusions however have not been used to establish 'laws', or to rule out conflicting explanations. They represent an 'open verdict' on what 'causes' anorexia and who typically suffers from it. As such they differ from the narrower, exclusive findings typical of most positivist research.

Positivist explanations are offered with a high degree of certainty. Clinicians deal in certainties because you often need them in order to take a specific action or do something about a problem (with uncertainty leading to inaction). But it is debatable whether such certitude genuinely increases our understanding of anorexia. Such explanations endeavour to unlock the secret of the disorder by discovering its key causes, but in so doing they tend to rule out alternative explanations. Even before any data have been gathered the terms of reference are to find a single answer to the question of what causes anorexia. By stating an hypothesis, e.g. 'anorexics come from middle class families', a tacit imperative to look for data to support the hypothesis tends to be incorporated into the study.

The results of my study tell us a great deal about anorexics. But they also tell us just as much about the way in which the psychiatric research community has constructed a model of the woman who gets anorexia. In constructing this model, psychiatrists focus on a particular group who are thus more likely to be diagnosed. In like manner many feminists have also constructed a stereotype of the anorexic as a political prisoner protesting against the injustices of patriarchy (Orbach, 1993). Psychiatrists however have produced a much larger body of empirical research on anorexia than feminists. The psychiatric stereotype, has therefore become the most powerful and pervasive image of the type of person likely to develop anorexia.

Psychiatry thus searches for 'certainty'. There is a great deal of evidence however (Hepworth, 1999, Scull, 1982, Showalter, 1987, Fisher, 2001, Kutchins and Kirk, 1997, Ussher, 1991) to suggest that far from being fixed and immutable, psychiatric diagnoses are fluid and evolve in response to changes in wider society. This may be the case in relation to the anorexic stereotype. It may well be that the current constructions that psychiatry places on the typical anorexic will evolve and develop over time. Such an evolutionary process is evident in relation to the development of psychiatric diagnoses over recent decades (Kutchins and Kirk, 1997). In the 1950s for example, consistent with prevailing social prejudices, homosexuality was considered a psychiatric illness (Kutchins and Kirk, 1997, Bayer, 1987). Later, in response to the changes in the status of gay men and women, such a diagnosis was abandoned.

Notwithstanding the changing nature of the diagnostic criteria applied to anorexia nervosa, psychiatrists continue to construct anorexia as a highly specific pathology with fixed diagnostic criteria. Part of this process of looking for certainty leads psychiatrists to direct their attention towards a specific demographic profile. It is not only in the demographic area, however, that a stereotype has been constructed. A stereotype of the anorexic's cognitive symptoms is also evident. Anorexics, psychiatrists suggest, exhibit distinct emotional symptoms, such as fear of maturity, fat phobia, control and obsessionalism. This book seeks to demonstrate that the cognitive model of the stereotypical anorexic is itself a social construction, developed by the psychiatric research community. As the next three chapters will demonstrate, the reality of who gets anorexia and of what causes it, is a great deal more complex than the cognitive model of the stereotype anorexic would suggest.

Chapter 6
'I am terrified of gaining weight': Results from the Closed-ended Cognitive Questionnaire

Introduction

This chapter (and Chapters 7 and 8) assess the validity of the cognitive stereotype of anorexia. In the first part of the chapter a brief review of this stereotype is presented. The chapter then describes the questionnaire which the current study used to appraise the symptoms in the cognitive stereotype, and it finally presents data from anorexics and controls gathered by this closed-ended questionnaire. As explained earlier, the cognitive stereotype constructs the anorexic as afraid of maturity. According to this paradigm anorexia represents a fear of full female adulthood and a flight from full genital sexuality. A corollary of this symptom is the notion of the 'anorexogenic' mother who has failed to prepare her child for the demands of adult life (Crisp, 1995). Crisp, a psychiatrist, explains:

> The mother [...] because she lacks a wider competence as a mother, may feed excessive amounts to her child as a substitute for her love and affection [...] The nervous over-protective mother who anxiously nurtures her child in this way so as to 'prepare him [sic] for the future' [...] may feel great anxiety over anything her child does outside her direct supervision and yet rarely attend to his differential cues [...] It appears to me that the importance of childhood experience for both the anorexic and her family is that it often in no way equips them to cope with the thrust and demands of puberty. (1995: 45–7)

Crisp therefore clearly identifies anorexia as a crisis of maturity. He lays the blame for this crisis squarely with the anorexic's mother. A critique of this mother-blaming approach is offered later (see Chapter 7). In the current chapter, the symptom associated with mother blaming, 'fear of maturity' is appraised. Such a symptom centres on 'maturational crises', while other symptoms incorporate a different focus. Most psychiatrists, for example stress the centrality of dieting to anorexia. In particular they emphasise 'weight phobia' (Buckroyd, 1996, Palmer, 1989). Palmer, for example, explains:

> Someone in a state of anorexia nervosa will not always be frank about her feelings, but when she is she will say that she is frightened of the thought of being heavier [...] Professor Crisp of St. George's Hospital Medical School, London, has coined the term 'weight phobia' to describe this attitude [...] the anorexic has a phobia of her normal body weight. (1989:5)

What is interesting about Palmer's observation is the manner in which the anorexic's state of mind is labelled. Highly technical and psychiatric terms are used, with her symptoms being described as 'phobia'. Buckroyd also describes anorexia as 'phobia' (1996:8,71) and stresses fear of fatness as central to the condition. At the beginning of her book, she quotes from one of her anorexic patients:

> Everyone in my class was going on a diet, so I did too, except that they all stopped and I didn't. To start with I was pleased. I felt proud that I had more willpower than they did, but in the end it was awful because I couldn't stop dieting. They had all lost a few pounds so that they could get into a size smaller dress, but I just went on and on. In the end I got so I was frightened to eat anything. In one part of my head I knew that I had to eat and that I needed to eat, but in another I thought I was fat and that if I ate anything it would make me fatter. (1996:3)

The focus on the anorexic's concern with 'anything' that would 'make me fatter' suggests that dieting and fat phobia, in Buckroyd's view, are two of the most important manifestations of anorexia. Other commentators have emphasised additional traits such as perfectionism (Russell, 1970, Garner et al, 1983b, Lawrence, 1995). Marilyn Lawrence (1995) explains that perfectionism manifests itself in self-denial, achieved through overcoming the physical demands of the flesh. 'We are all encouraged to regard self-denial as a good thing' because 'the ability to limit food and to lose weight bring with them a far-reaching moral kudos' (1995:33).

Clinical understanding of anorexia therefore presents the disorder as fat phobia and maturity fear, experienced by perfectionist personalities. A further and equally important area of the 'cognitive stereotype' is the symptom of control. Lawrence explains that 'the obsessional aspect of anorexia is without a doubt a desperate need to be in control' (1995:23), while Strober (1980) suggests that a need for control is the key feature of anorexia. The importance of control is emphasised by almost every commentator on the disorder (Palmer, 1989, Orbach, 1993, Bruch, 1979, Crisp, 1995, Buckroyd, 1996, Levenkron, 2000) and this construct, I feel, genuinely applies to many anorexic patients (see Chapter 7).

In this chapter, I will appraise the 'cognitive stereotype'. The symptoms surrounding this stereotype form a key element in closed-ended rating instruments applied to anorexia (Garner et al, 1983b). One such instrument is the Eating Disorders Inventory (EDI, Garner et al, 1983b). In the current study, an adapted version of the EDI, (the EDI-A, see Appendix) was administered to a sub-sample of 24 anorexic patients and all 100 controls.

The Adapted EDI (EDI-A)

The Eating Disorders Inventory is an important clinical questionnaire used in anorexia research (Garner et al, 1983b). It closely reflects the 'clinical' model of anorexia, and thus contains several 'attitude statement' questions on 'fat phobia' and 'fear of maturity'. Examples of these questions are:

> I am terrified of gaining weight
> I am pre-occupied with the desire to be thinner
> I wish I could return to the security of childhood
> I would rather be an adult than a child

As well as containing questions on fat phobia and maturity fear, the schedule also contains questions on perfectionism. The following statements cover this item:

Only outstanding performance is good enough in my family
I hate being less than best at things

In addition, the schedule measures control, by asking about feelings of 'ineffectiveness'. These are measured by the questions below:

I have a low opinion about myself
I feel ineffective as a person

In response to these questions patients are invited to tick one of the following:

	Always	Usually	Often	Sometimes	Rarely	Never
I have a low opinion about myself	( )	( )	( )	( )	( )	( )

The EDI specifies several key dimensions in the development of anorexia. For the current study, the dimensions which are of specific interest are 'Drive for Thinness', 'Maturity fears', 'Ineffectiveness' and 'Perfectionism'.[1] In relation to 'Drive for thinness' Garner et al state:

> Drive for thinness [...] indicates excessive concern with dieting, [and] pre-occupation with weight [...] Bruch (1973, 1978) and others have described this as a cardinal feature of anorexia nervosa. Items [in the 'Drive for thinness' dimension] reflect both an ardent wish to lose weight as well as a fear of weight gain. (1983b:17)

Thus as Garner et al demonstrate, 'Drive for Thinness' in the 'classical' clinical view, is one of the most important dimensions for assessing anorexia nervosa. The EDI schedule therefore begins with

1 Items from other dimensions (see Appendix) were however also retained in order to administer the EDI in as close a format as possible to the original instrument.

questions on terror of weight gain, and it is this dimension which is discussed at the outset in accounts of the construction of the EDI (Garner et al, 1983b). Like 'Drive for thinness', 'Maturity fear' is similarly considered as central to the disorder:

> Maturity fears [...] indicate [a] wish to retreat to the security of [childhood and a fear of] [...] the overwhelming demands of adulthood. (Garner et al, 1983b:17–19)

This symptom features centrally in the EDI and is thus considered one of the key manifestations of anorexia nervosa. Similarly the dimension 'Ineffectiveness' is also felt to encapsulate a key causative factor in the genesis of the illness. As stated above, the 'Ineffectiveness' dimension illustrates the importance of loss of control in the development of anorexia. As Garner et al (1983b) explain:

> Ineffectiveness [...] assesses feelings of general inadequacy [...] and the feeling of not being in control of one's life. This feature has been described by some as the fundamental disturbance in anorexia nervosa. (Garner et al, 1983b18)

Loss of control is therefore considered pivotal to anorexic aetiology. A further symptom also viewed as central to the disorder is the symptom of perfectionism:

> Perfectionism [...] indicates excessive personal expectations for superior achievement. Bruch (1978) has suggested that the struggle to live up to perfectionistic achievement standards is a characteristic theme in anorexia nervosa. She interprets the patient's typical superior academic performance as an 'over-compliant adaptation' which breaks down in the face of increasing pressures to succeed. (Garner et al, 1983b:18)

Clearly, since the EDI is an important clinical instrument applied to anorexia , (see e.g. Cantrell and Ellis, 1991, Heebink et al, 1995, Taylor et al, 1996, Sands et al, 1997), and since its questions encapsulate the clinical model of the disorder, it was important to establish whether the EDI-A was able to discriminate between anorexics and controls on the above four dimensions. Results from the 'Drive for thinness', 'Maturity fears', 'Ineffectiveness', and 'Perfectionism' dimensions, together with results from the global EDI-A score will now be presented.

Results from the EDI-A

For EDI-A items, a global score was calculated from results from all of the questions asked. For each question, where participants answered 'always', 'usually' or 'often', a score of 1 was given. Where participants answered 'sometimes', 'rarely' or 'never', the item was scored as 0. A cut-off score of 20 (out of 30) was assigned (see page 79). This ensured that participants would need to affirm at least two thirds of the questions to exhibit symptoms clinicians identify as indicative of anorexia. A chi-square was also calculated to examine whether significant differences were observed between the answers supplied by the anorexics and the answers supplied by the controls. Using this scheme, the following results were obtained (table 6.1):

Table 6.1: Scores on the Adapted EDI – Anorexic and Control Subjects

	Anorexics	Controls
20 or more questions affirmed	2	2
Less than 20 questions affirmed	22	98
Total	24	100

$\chi 2 =$ 2.487 df (1) (not significant)

These results indicate that, in the current study, the adapted EDI questionnaire failed to discriminate between a sample of anorexics and a sample of healthy controls. In other words healthy people were almost as likely as anorexics to affirm or deny a selection of questions from the EDI inventory.

This book aims to appraise the 'stereotypical' clinical construction of anorexia, which emphasises fear of fatness, fear of maturity, loss of control, and perfectionism. It was therefore important to examine the EDI's ability to discriminate (between anorexics and controls) on items from EDI dimensions that corresponded to these symptoms. The following items were selected from each dimension, and results on these items were compared for the anorexic and control group:

> Drive for thinness – items:
> 'I am terrified of gaining weight'
> 'I am pre-occupied with the desire to be thinner'
> Fear of maturity – item:
> 'I would rather be an adult than a child'
> Perfectionism – item:
> 'Only outstanding performance is good enough in my family'
> Ineffectiveness – items:
> 'I feel ineffective as a person'
> 'I have a low opinion about myself'

On two of these dimensions, 'maturity fears' and 'perfectionism', no significant differences were observed between the anorexic and control group for any of the items measured. For example, the item 'I would rather be an adult than a child', (table 6.2), was affirmed by 10 out of 24 anorexics, and 58 out of 100 controls. The chi-square statistic of 2.685 which was calculated for this item, was well below significance at the 5% level. Similarly, for the item 'only outstanding performance is good enough in my family' (from the perfectionism dimension), no significant differences between anorexics and controls were observed (table 6.3).

Table 6.2: Results from Anorexics and Controls on the EDI item: 'I would rather be an adult than a child' from the 'Maturity fears' dimension

	Anorexics	Controls
Yes	10	58
No	14	42
Total	24	100

$\chi 2 =$ 2.685 df(1) (not significant)

Table 6.3: Results from Anorexics and Controls on the EDI item: 'Only outstanding performance is good enough in my family' from the 'Perfectionism' dimension		
	Anorexics	Controls
Yes	8	22
No	16	78
Total	24	100

$\chi 2 =$ 1.355 df (1) (not significant)

Table 6.4: Results from Anorexics and Controls on the EDI item: 'I am terrified of gaining weight' from the 'Drive for thinness' dimension		
	Anorexics	Controls
Yes	23	35
No	1	65
Total	24	100

$\chi 2 =$ 28.770 df (1) (significant)

Table 6.5: Results from Anorexics and Controls on the EDI item: 'I am pre-occupied with the desire to be thinner' from the 'Drive for thinness' dimension		
	Anorexics	Controls
Yes	20	24
No	4	76
Total	24	100

$\chi 2 =$ 29.764 df (1) (significant)

The remaining dimensions that were of interest in the current study were the dimensions of 'Drive for Thinness' and 'Ineffectiveness'. On these dimensions significant differences were observed in the responses of anorexics when compared to controls (see Tables 6.4, 6.5, 6.6, and 6.7). Significant differences, for example, were observed for the item 'I am terrified of gaining weight'. This item however pertained to a highly corporeal aspect of the patient's condition. It is logical that when comparing anorexics with healthy women, fewer of the latter would report 'terror of gaining weight'. Such statistical significance however does not imply this item is the central feature of anorexia nervosa (though the DSM (APA, 1980, 1994) does imply this). Also, this question may have uncovered the outward manifestations of the disorder (which were bound to have been more fully evinced in anorexics when compared to controls) but it did not capture the complex underlying pre-cursors which may lead to these fat phobic symptoms. The one dimension which did attempt to uncover more complex 'causes' was the dimension 'Ineffectiveness'. This dimension measured feelings of loss of control on the part of the patient. Highly significant differences were observed between the anorexic and the control group for this dimension. For the two items 'I feel ineffective as a person' and 'I have a low opinion about myself' the responses supplied by anorexic and control subjects were as follows:

Table 6.6: Results from Anorexics and Controls for the EDI item: 'I feel ineffective as a person' from the 'Ineffectiveness' dimension

	Anorexics	Controls
Yes	19	7
No	5	93
Total	24	100

$\chi 2 =$ 60.828 df (1) (significant)

Table 6.7: Results from Anorexics and Controls for the EDI item: 'I have a low opinion about myself' from the 'Ineffectiveness' dimension

	Anorexics	Controls
Yes	23	17
No	1	83
Total	24	100

$\chi 2 =$ 55.044 df (1) (significant)

The overall trend in results from the EDI-A showed fairly modest ability to discriminate between the anorexics and controls in the study.

While some of the items in the EDI-A showed good ability to discriminate, particularly on the 'ineffectiveness' dimension, the ability of the instrument to 'uncover' anorexia in the current sample was limited. Differences in the global EDI-A scores between the groups were not significant and differences between the scores for the two groups on several individual items also failed to reach significance levels.

The results from the adapted EDI are especially illuminating when we consider that the instrument clearly encapsulates the clinical stereotype of what 'causes' anorexia. From the outset, by asking a series of questions on terror of weight gain, the EDI underlines the clinical importance attached to this particular symptom, and identifies fat phobia as one of the key manifestations of the illness, rather than (as the current study argues) as an outcome of much more deep seated social and psychological pre-cursors. Fat phobia therefore remains privileged as the key criterion for anorexia nervosa. Also, by incorporating questions on maturity fears and perfectionism, the EDI further underlines the clinical tendency to construct the anorexic as a perfectionist, high achiever, retreating from the pressures of independent adulthood. For these items also however the difference in the answers provided by anorexics and controls in the current study were not significant.

In appraising the EDI's potential to show only limited ability to discriminate between anorexic and control participants, Garner et al assert that:

> like all self-report instruments, the EDI is vulnerable to distortion due to response style bias and inaccurate reporting by the subject. Moreover the defensive structure of the patient may invalidate or distort self-evaluation data. (1983b:32)

According to Garner et al, where the EDI fails to clearly specify cases of anorexia (as in the current study), this has resulted from the withholding of information by the patient, for defensive reasons. Similarities in EDI responses between anorexics and controls, Garner et al imply, are artefactual rather than real. I disagree with this suggestion and feel there is a more fundamental explanation. The patient's illness, I feel, may have resulted from experiences outside of those covered in the EDI. Some of these experiences may be social in nature. It is notable, for example that almost all anorexics are women. Notwithstanding the gains of feminism, however, present day culture remains essentially masculinist. This is evidenced in the continued exclusion of women from high paid jobs, (Callender, 1996), high profile government positions, and in the continuing failure to prioritise women centred social policy in the area of childcare and domestic violence (Hallet, 1996). The disempowerment which women may consequently feel might have contributed to the growth of anorexia. By demarcating a limited psycho-social profile as the territory of anorexia, the EDI tends to ignore these (possibly equally valid) explanations. It also fails to acknowledge the problematic relationship all women arguably have with food (Lawrence, 1995, Orbach, 1993). Most women, at some point in their lives, may well have felt 'terrified of gaining weight' or 'preoccupied with the desire to be thinner'.

Despite its limitations, the EDI remains one of the most important clinical and research instruments for assessing anorexia (see e.g. Cantrell and Ellis, 1991, Heebink et al, 1995, Taylor et al, 1996, Sands et al, 1997). Indeed two patients in the current sample reported that they had been administered the EDI in the past[2]. When asked to state their feelings about the questionnaire, it was interesting that patients' answers were varied. While some patients appeared to feel that the questionnaire was almost uncannily prescient, and described their experiences exactly, others expressed frustration that the questionnaire appeared to focus on cosmetic dieting behaviour. Some participants even felt that the questionnaire was irrelevant, inaccurate and irritating.

Ann[3] for example, felt the questionnaire was interesting. Her main response was surprise at how the researchers appeared to know so much about her own experience and the factors that had led up to

2 This may arguably have led to a practice effect (where patients pre-empt the answers 'expected' having completed the EDI before). However such an effect might have been expected to persuade patients to affirm the EDI's questions thus increasing their scores when compared to the scores of controls. In the current study however, reasonable similarity was observed in scores between controls and anorexics.

3 To maintain confidentiality, pseudonyms have been given to patients.

her illness. Rachel and Gail also felt the questionnaire was relevant, and Christine, Lucy and Paula found the questionnaire similarly straightforward and stimulating. Some patients however, (such as John, Samantha, Tracy, Barbara and Genevive) had mixed or even negative feelings. John felt the questionnaire was not at all related to his illness, while Samantha felt it was 'totally wide of the mark'. Another patient, Tracey, was even conscious of the questionnaire's tendency to 'over-categorise' patients. 'In a way', she suggested, 'I think some of [the questions] are sort of set to put you in a sort of box [...] as a [...] typical anorexic or bulimic'. On the whole, participants gave a mixture of responses when asked to state their opinions about the questionnaire they had just been administered.

Patients' feelings about the EDI were thus inconclusive, as were the results from many of the EDI items. The key conclusions which we may draw from the data presented in this chapter are that a highly circumscribed clinical instrument may fail to fully discriminate between anorexics and 'healthy' women. There may thus be other reasons for anorexia than those laid down in this instrument. It may also be the case that, while some anorexics experience certain symptoms, others do not. By identifying a rigid template, clinicians are potentially doing a disservice to patients. They may fail to engage with the specific causes of the patient's illness which may be outside the criteria laid down in this template. By privileging a limited number of symptoms as central to anorexia, clinicians may be in danger of over-valuing these symptoms. They may thus be prone to interpret patient's experiences to fit this symptom template, selecting those aspects of patients' accounts which conform to the clinical model, while relegating those which do not to a position of lesser importance.

The EDI-A illustrated the current state of clinical thinking about anorexia. As such it provided an excellent template by which the nature of clinical 'knowledge' surrounding anorexia may be gauged. If such knowledge is incontestable and unproblematic then the results gathered by such an instrument should clearly discriminate between a group of anorexics and a group of controls. The fact that in this study they did not raises important questions about the nature of clinical thought surrounding the illness. As sociologists it is important to present these results with a view to arguing that such inconsistencies underscore the sociological contention that knowledge categories are arrived at through a process of negotiation between powerful groups (Burke, 2000, Berger and Luckman, 1966), and may not always reflect the experience of every patient. This has important implications for the general argument in the current study and an account of the importance of these findings for the overall thesis will now be offered.

Conclusion: Importance of the EDI-A Findings for the Overall Thesis

The study aims to investigate clinical knowledge surrounding anorexia. It aims to assess whether the 'stereotype' of the anorexic as an appearance obsessed youngster who is afraid to grow up is supported by data. In the current chapter, I appraise the cognitive stereotype of the anorexic. According to the results in this chapter, this cognitive stereotype may have limited data to support it. Notwithstanding the small size of the sample, (and the subsequent limitations in the validity of the study's results), the current chapter appears to give an initial indication that elements of the cognitive stereotype are not always supported by data.

A key element of the cognitive stereotype is 'maturity fear'. The anorexic, it is argued, (Crisp, 1995), is recoiling from adult femininity, and from the responsibilities that this role brings. Many patients in the current study, however, denied that they were afraid of maturity. Nevertheless, the archetype of the anorexic as an adolescent girl retreating from feminine adulthood and full genital sexuality remains one of the clearest and most persistent images of anorexia (Bruch, 1978, Crisp, 1995). It is thus important to examine why fear of maturity continues to form a key part of the clinical model. Clinical understanding reflects sexist constructions of 'female' illnesses (Ussher, 1991). By emphasising 'fear of maturity' clinicians constitute anorexics as recalcitrant adolescents fleeing from adulthood. That their anorexia may be an understandable response to the injustices of their lives is not considered. Instead their unhappiness is constructed as a deficiency on the part of the sufferer.

Clinical knowledge thus reflects a patriarchal definition of the 'causes' of anorexia. Such a definition oppresses women on two fronts. Firstly it trivialises women's pain and categorises it under stereotypical labels such as 'maturity fear'. Secondly such a model fails to recognise that where anorexics do experience 'fear of maturity' they are fleeing from a debased, second-class identity. It is the role of adult femininity that is unhealthy and the behaviour of the anorexic is simply an understandable refusal to accept a sub-ordinate social position.

Anorexia is also identified as a strategy of control (Lawrence, 1995). This symptom was clearly supported by the data in this chapter, with patients suggesting that they felt 'ineffective'. Clinical explanations however tend to ignore the wider social causes of women's disempowerment which lead to 'ineffectiveness'. If anorexia is about loss of control than the social forces which underpin women's disempowerment should be a central focus in the study of the illness. These social forces may be located in the discrimination women experience at work, their experience of unequal power at home (which may culminate in domestic violence) and in their location as 'second-class' citizens in wider society.

Rather than addressing these social forces, current clinical knowledge tends to cite individual family dynamics (Bruch, 1978, Minuchin, 1991) or trauma in the life of the individual patient (Palmer et al, 1990) as 'causing' the disorder. While these individual experiences are undoubtedly important, little attempt is made to theorise the unequal power relations that give rise to these traumas, and scant attention is given to the wider social structures, such as institutionalised patriarchy, through which this power imbalance is maintained.

Control (and 'fear of maturity') are therefore central to the clinical model. Such a model incorporates a further symptom – the symptom of fat phobia. Fat phobia underscores the clinical focus on bodily concerns. The current study however argues that anorexia is about more than just bodily concerns, and that fat phobia and dieting for reasons of appearance are secondary to psychological issues in the development of the illness. Feminists have explained that constructs such as fear of fatness may represent 'normal' emotions and describe experiences which all women have with food (Lawrence, 1995, Orbach, 1993). By re-packaging such symptoms as clinical phenomena, physicians render these 'normal' emotions in technical terms, and the common sense everyday attitudes of ordinary life are subordinated to the technical constructions of clinical knowledge.

The current chapter provides a clear illustration of clinical knowledge surrounding anorexia. It describes the manner in which the patient is prompted by a questionnaire to consider her illness in 'clinicalised' terms. However, many patients in the current study did not affirm these clinical symptoms. In rejecting these constructs, patients were indirectly questioning the legitimacy of medical definitions of their illness. It is evident from the results described in this chapter that patients' experiences may be wider than the clinical model would suggest. By attending to these wider experiences clinicians may effect a more understanding appraisal of the patient's condition. As a result, patients may be more likely to experience a feeling of being understood. Such an experience has been identified as an important indicator of the success (or otherwise) of treatment (Hsu et al, 1992).

On a wider level also, such a 'patient-centred' approach may better accommodate an understanding of the general social issues, which may lead to anorexia. Where clinicians focus on dieting and appearance, the real disadvantages and biases which women experience (in the home, in the workplace and in society) may be disregarded, along with the experience of disempowerment such disadvantages bring. By focussing largely on cosmetic issues, clinicians may be failing to evaluate patients' real concerns – concerns that arise from the real and complex lived experience of being ill in the social world.

In the next two chapters, patients' testimonies gathered in the open-ended interviews (conducted after the questionnaire was administered) are analysed. As we shall see, these testimonies broadly corroborate the responses which patients supplied to the closed-ended questionnaire. In the open-ended interview patients expressed dissatisfaction with the representation of anorexia as a disorder that chiefly centred on cosmetic concerns. In the patients' view, as evidenced in their narratives, much more complex factors had led to their disorder. It is to a discussion of these issues that I now turn.

Chapter 7
'Why I won't eat': Detailed Testimony from Anorexic Patients concerning the Causes of their Disorder

Introduction

In Chapter 6, I argued that women may have all kinds of reasons for developing anorexia and that these reasons may not always be reflected in 'stereotypical' definitions of the disorder. As well as analysing closed-ended data, the study also collected open-ended narratives from a sub sample of 24 anorexics (three male), to assess the importance of fat phobia, fear of maturity, control and perfectionism in 'causing' the illness. Patients were asked a simple question 'What would you say were the causes of your anorexia?' In response, patients were invited to talk for as long as they wished on subjects that they felt were relevant. This chapter describes the data collected in this open-ended interview. Initially, it outlines the manner in which the data were analysed (using thematic analysis, Hewitt-Taylor, 2001). It then presents a summary of the themes which emerged from the open ended-data, and finally it presents examples of the transcripts from which the themes were generated.

Patient testimony suggested that the causes ascribed to anorexia were varied. The data gathered in these open-ended accounts were therefore as diverse as the data on education, place of residence and social class (see Chapter 5). The patients had been referred from several geographical areas, and significant variation was observed in terms of their appearance, emotionality, and speech patterns. Some patients for example were talkative and voluble, while others were extremely quiet and difficult to draw out. A number of patients had a 'working class' (Bernstein, 1971) vernacular, (with words and sentences punctuated with phrases such as, 'you know, like', and 'you know what I mean'), while the speech patterns of others were unmistakably middle class. Several patients appeared anxious to please the interviewer and to acquiesce to anything they felt she might say, while others appeared more ready for a confrontation, wherein they would put the record straight on the 'genuine causes' of anorexia nervosa. In general, patients appeared to be a visibly diverse group from a range of different social strata.

Coding the Interview Data using Thematic Analysis

Participants were asked the following open-ended question – 'What would you say were the causes of your anorexia?' The data gathered in response to this question were analysed using thematic analysis (Hewitt-Taylor, 2001). This approach describes a process whereby I conducted a thorough examination of the patient transcripts and selected the key themes which encapsulated patient's experience. Such a process was facilitated by the use of the NU.DIST data analysis package (Gahan and Hannibal, 1998).

This was a time of reflection where I read and re-read patients' testimonies and sifted and appraised the content of patient accounts. This process resulted in the production of a key category, 'becoming anorexic'. 'Becoming anorexic' involved two phases. These phases were 'not being anorexic' and 'being anorexic'. The variations in patients' progression towards anorexia were explained by describing experiences that determined movement from one phase into another. The category 'becoming anorexic' identified the nexus of the research and represented an inclusive category under which all sub-categories could be classified. This category could not be subsumed under any other category, but all sub-categories could be integrated into it.

In addition to the core category, two sub-categories 'trigger' and 'sustain' were also produced (see figure 7.1). The sub-category 'trigger' described the process through which participants moved from a state of not being an anorexic into being an anorexic. The maintenance of the state of anorexia such that the patient may be said to have truly become an anorexic is encapsulated by the sub-category 'sustain'. Under both 'trigger' and 'sustain' most patients in the sample reported significant issues in relation to almost all of the categories identified.

Coding the data

The categories under 'trigger' and 'sustain' were identified via a process of coding (Hewitt-Taylor 2001, Bowling, 1997, Strauss and Corbin, 1990). Coding involved a thorough appraisal of transcripts to identify the issues of concern to patients. Words and lines were closely scrutinised, and categories were thus allocated using the exact wording of the patients themselves. The meanings of these concepts to the sample of patients were therefore fully encapsulated in the category labels. Using this technique the following categories were identified:

Diverse experiences have caused my anorexia
Anorexia is complex
Unhappiness
Family
Life Event
School
Control
The Buzz
The Spiral
Obsessionalism/perfectionism
Anorexia is not just slimming

The first theme to be identified was the theme 'diverse experiences have caused my anorexia'. This theme, together with the text from which it was generated, will now be discussed.

Figure 7.1 ‘Becoming Anorexic’

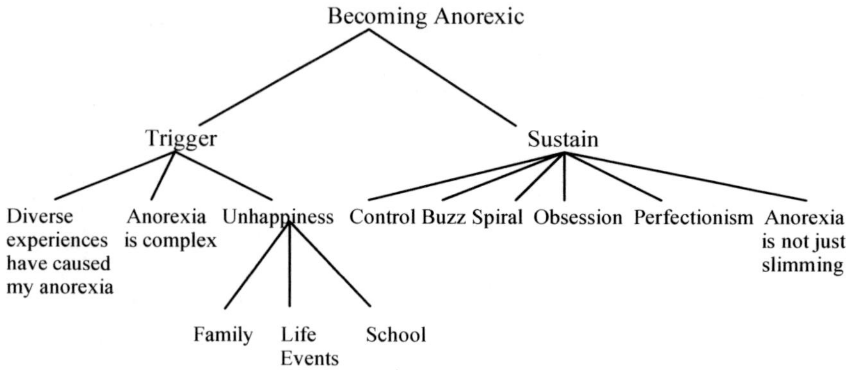

Figure 7.1 ‘Becoming Anorexic’

Table 7.1: The Triggers and ‘Causes’ of Anorexia	
(from n= 24 respondents)	Number of respondents citing trigger
Diverse experiences have caused my anorexia	12
Anorexia is complex	11
Unhappiness	16
Family	15
Life Event	14
School	8
Control	20
The Buzz	15
The Spiral	7
Obsessionalism/perfectionism	11
Anorexia is not just slimming	15

NB: Respondents could identify more than one trigger/cause

'Diverse experiences have caused my anorexia'

Several patients identified a specific life event which was important in the development of their illness. What was interesting about these events however was not their similarity, but rather the diverse nature of the events each patient described.[1] The first participant to tell her story was Rachel. Rachel explained that the roots of her anorexia could be traced to the events surrounding her mother and natural-father's separation when she was a toddler. A series of highly painful episodes associated with this occurrence had shaped Rachel's early life. In spite of the good care she received from her mother, she continued to be affected by this. When she was a child, her father's family had sought custody of her. By involving child care agencies, her father had attempted to brand her mother as unfit:

> there was an awful lot of that that I absorbed. I wasn't you know returned to my father … but er I've noticed now whenever I get depressed I naturally don't want to eat.

As part of her testimony, Rachel described an event which occurred shortly after her mother's divorce. Rachel's mother re-married, and Rachel discovered that her stepfather was not her natural father. Though her stepfather was an excellent parent, this news about her background troubled Rachel. She was gripped by an intense longing to know who her natural father really was. The news about her parentage:

> set up burning questions you know ... 'who is my real father?' and why mother didn't want me to find out nothing about him – she felt it was water under the bridge best forgotten about, but to me, that was that dreadful ... I didn't want to hurt my stepfather … but still all the while there's that nagging, you know.

These experiences in Rachel's view, had a material effect on the development of her illness. She was intensely concerned about the

1 For the purposes of confidentiality I have disguised some of the details in these highly individualised accounts.

damage which had been inflicted on her mother, and shouldered the responsibility of wanting to put things right. Rachel described herself as extremely influenced by the hard life her mother had endured.

> I wanted to be doing all the right things [for my mother], to be ... as perfect as I possibly could – I think ... I set myself too high a standard ... I had to strive.

This perfectionism later manifested itself in an obsessional adherence to diets, eventually leading to anorexia nervosa.

Other participants also supplied detailed accounts of why they had become anorexic. Unlike Rachel, Angela had a very close relationship with her natural father. When he sadly died Angela could no longer face food:

> Well ... me dad was so ill and ... I couldn't ... handle him dying cos like we had to look after him at home cos he was dying of cancer ... it just affected me that I felt like ... cos I was underweight I felt like it should be me that's ... dying and not him – because like I'd ... done it to myself whereas he obviously didn't ... have a choice ... it just sort of affected me where ... I just didn't want to eat. It just sort of affected me that ... I didn't deserve really to ... live.

As a result of this trauma, Angela's intake of food almost completely ceased. She rapidly lost weight, eventually plummeting to five and a half stones. Once she started to lose the weight, she 'felt very good about it so y'know I sort of continued it and I loved it'. The experience of bereavement had propelled Angela into involuntary weight loss from which she derived unanticipated pleasure.

Other patients described different circumstances. John for example had been very lonely as a boy. The sense of inadequacy he thus experienced was aggravated by persistent teasing and bullying from age mates. This caused John to engage in a constant search for admiration and approval. The congratulatory remarks he received after successfully dieting immediately precipitated a period of anorexia. Like John, Genevive also identified complex life events which 'caused' her disorder. Genevive felt that her experience of being sent to boarding school during her adolescence was a major trigger in the onset of her illness. This trigger, however, had combined with others to produce a complex picture. As child, for example, Genevive had been moved from town to town because of her father's work and the disruption she thus experienced had contributed to her anorexia. Like many patients, Genevive clearly believed that anorexia was a very complicated disorder. This point was reiterated by patient after patient, and it is to a discussion of the complex nature of anorexia nervosa that we now turn.

'Anorexia is complex'

Patients supplied a rich variety of reasons for their illness. As we have seen, many were aware that the disorder had complex origins and could not be accounted for by reference to a single pre-cursor. As one patient explained, 'it's complicated', a sentiment which was echoed by many other patients. Participant after participant clearly identified the puzzling nature of anorexia nervosa. Lucy suggested 'I think a lot of things probably had an effect ... it's something that is ... very much misunderstood'. Similarly, Samantha reported that it was 'very, very difficult' to explain her self-starvation:

> it doesn't seem logical at all, it seems very warped even though I do it to myself ... and it's very difficult to explain why you do it, but I just feel good when I'm doing it to myself so that's how I cope.

Rachel also believed that anorexia was a baffling and complex disorder. Rachel explained that the different episodes of anorexia she had experienced over the years had different causes. 'I'm really struggling now', she suggested 'because this time has been different from any other time'. When asked what influenced the onset of her illness in the first place, she replied that that was a difficult question to answer. Whether one became anorexic, Rachel believed, depended on the type of person one was and one's ability to cope with life.

Anorexia was thus described as 'complicated'. Some patients suggested that society over-simplified the disorder, and this made them angry. Emma expressed frustration at society's tendency to view the disorder in simplistic terms. She felt that the illness was so complex 'that it makes me angry when people try and put it in boxes and ... try and generalise and stuff'. This frustration was echoed by other patients including John, Richard, Samantha and Lucy. Lucy believed that anorexia was a response to many different sorts of unhappiness. The factors which could 'cause' the illness were complex and intertwined, which could generate internal confusion. Ann, for example, explained:

> lots of things were happening around me, people kept going at me and picking on me and … I just felt out of control then I think – I just didn't know what was happening to me … I was just changing, everything was changing, my personality was changing.

Genevive also suggested that she did not know what 'any one thing' had singly caused her anorexia, and Julie also believed that the effects of the trauma she experienced had combined with other stresses to produce the illness. Julie had survived serious abuse in childhood, but even in the face of such adversity, she felt that other factors (albeit to a lesser degree) had also helped cause her condition. Anorexia, in Julie's view, could therefore be caused by any number of stresses, an opinion echoed by Angela. In Angela's interview the following insight was offered into why anorexia develops:

> Angela: I think it's just anything really like you know if you've been abused or anything in your childhood or ... didn't have a really good upbringing I think it just affects you
>
> Interviewer: Why?
>
> Angela: I don't know. I don't know about that. I think it's just ... anything really.
>
> Interviewer: So you're saying anything traumatic can make you …
>
> Angela: Oh yeah, yeah. depression can put you off food and then you just get into a routine of not eating and then you know you probably like yourself as you lose weight, so it just keeps, you know, it just goes out of control.

Other patients' testimonies reinforced this causative complexity. Lucy, for example was asked whether anorexia was a 'control' or a 'cosmetic' strategy. Her reply; 'I'd say it was probably a bit of both', once more illustrated the multi-layered nature of the disorder. This complexity was reflected in the very sophisticated explanations which some patients gave for the cause of their illness. One such explanation was supplied by Barbara who reported that she liked to get attention and admiration. At a particular stage in her adolescence Barbara no longer felt her achievements were sufficient for her to obtain the admiration she so badly craved. She could no longer:

> get the attention by being good in my own right and I ... started to focus on food ... my eating disorder ... was something that I could do when I couldn't face up to life. [It allowed me] to really engage with something because I feel I'm alone in the world completely. I mean I often feel scared of doing anything because I'm scared I'll fail ... I'm scared of doing anything like reading or ... engaging with anything external – I know it sounds quite mad really but ... when I binge ... that's simple ... it's one thing that I can really absorb myself into and sometimes I feel dead inside – you know I used to be passionate about things but nowadays I feel just dead. When I feel like that – I feel like the food is one thing that gets me sort of passionate again because I can sort of absorb myself and be angry – it's like screaming and crying you know just an extreme emotion when you're bingeing and then an extreme emotion when you're purging ... you know I want my life to be perfect straight away. Life takes too long to sort out ... but eating – I mean it makes you feel instantly better ... what you really want to do is ... sort [out] your life but it's impossible to do that ... so you ... put [your aspirations] on top of the food ... it's a way of realising aspirations and dreams that are impossible.

Barbara's lucid testimony movingly conveys many patients' motivations for becoming anorexic. These patients were very clear about the profoundly complex nature of their illness. They understood that its causes and the strategy they might adopt for recovery, were diverse. John, for example, adopted a highly personal strategy for recovery, involving a resolution to address the underlying source of his pathology. This would incorporate a determined focus on building his self-esteem and finding new ways of liking himself. While John showed self-awareness in adopting this approach, he was uncertain how successful this strategy would be:

> once I get out [unless] I sort my head out ... and get myself with more self-esteem and respect for myself there's nothing to say that … all the weight I've put on [won't] all come off again. Unless I ... actually feel as though ... I'm good at something ... and I can go and achieve something and ... feel positive and ... do things that I ... want to do in my life ... then I feel as though I will always turn to food to ... get the good feelings.

'Unhappiness'

One of the key themes to emerge from the open-ended data was the theme of unhappiness. Something had gone wrong in the lives of these anorexic patients. This unhappiness may have been the result of a traumatic event such as bereavement, an experience of being bullied at school, or a history of sexual or physical abuse. Equally however, the dysfunction in patients' lives frequently resulted from more diffuse and long term negative experiences. One patient, Lucy, for example, explained the generalised sense of loss she experienced because she felt she had never really been important in the life of her parents. While her parents conveyed high expectations, they were less exact about precisely what it was they did expect. If she performed well in school, her parents' reaction was 'that's what we expect of you'. She consequently felt she had never developed a proper relationship with them, either as a child or an adult. Another patient, John, explained that while his parents were loving, because of work they failed to spend much time with him. 'Mum and Dad ... put a lot of time into the business ... they did their very best for me certainly, but ... I wanted more time with them which I didn't get'.

This sense of unhappiness had often become distilled into a profound sense of dissatisfaction, on the part of the patient with the way she or he looked. Many patients expressed unhappiness with their appearance, and a smaller number described this dissatisfaction as centring on their weight. In spite of several prompts to discuss weight issues, however, several patients were very clear that their dissatisfaction with their appearance was part of a generalised sense of unhappiness, and was not centred purely on feeling fat.

Other patients experienced a sense of dissatisfaction and loss as a result of their experiences at school. Several described a failure to fit in, particularly at secondary school. One woman explained that she had always felt out of place. She felt inadequate and was constantly comparing herself to other girls in her class. For others, this sense of being an outsider was frequently accompanied by being teased, bullied and passed over. Gail explained that as a result of an argument with an age-mate she was harassed and excluded by the whole of her class, while John explained 'I got a lot of ... bullying and ... at school I'd get called fatty.' Yet another patient. Paula, was bullied jointly by siblings and school mates:

> When I was younger I used to get bullied a lot for being fat ... they used to call me names and everything ... It was em when I was in secondary school ... it just went on through most of school ... even me own sisters used to pick on me for being fat ... my friends would join in and make fun out of me as well ... they made fun of me cos they could always get a boyfriend when they went out and I couldn't.

What is interesting in these accounts is that victims were not abused by the archetypal 'school bully'. None were 'picked on' in the schoolyard or divested of their money with menaces on their way home. These youngsters were bullied instead by large groups of 'popular' schoolgirls. From these transcripts one was left with the impression that the perpetrators of this abuse were well integrated into the school system. The abuse was based not around physical violence, but rather on 'pointedly' nasty remarks and 'backbiting'. It was nevertheless equally aggressive and damaging to the victim's self-esteem. Already often rendered powerless by familial abuse, victims were singled out for further harassment. In cases like this, the bullies were in the majority and the victim in a minority of one.

Regardless of whether bullying was involved, negative experiences of some form in the lives of these anorexic patients had given rise to a great sense of pain and loss. All were unhappy. Phrases like 'low in confidence', 'shy' 'unhappy' and lacking in 'self-esteem' were frequently uttered during the course of the interviews. As Ann explained 'I'm quite sort of depressed and I keep crying all the time and I'm low in myself', while Rachel described how her anorexia always seemed to return during periods of depression.

Perhaps unsurprisingly this generalised sense of unhappiness was echoed in the unhappiness patients experienced over the way they looked. 'I just didn't like the way I looked', Ann remarked, 'I was unhappy really'. This sense of body dissatisfaction however did not seem to diminish as the patient became slimmer. No matter how thin she became, the patient still appeared to want to lose more weight. Angela summarised this succinctly, 'I know five and a half stone is low but I'm not happy now with the way I am. I want to be a lot less.' Because of their sense of unhappiness, several respondents explained that there was a gap in their lives. Lucy described this as an 'unhappiness gap':

> perhaps the person like myself who kind of gets hooked into [anorexia] had a gap that needed filling ... because ... that gave me something to fill the gap ... whereas probably ... other people don't necessarily have one. [U]nhappiness ... perhaps it's as simple as that ... perhaps it's something to plug an unhappiness gap ... to prevent you ... I don't know ... but it just seems to me like something that plugs a gap – with control.

The notion of control is key to this extract. Participants adopted a strategy of rigid control over food to address the unhappiness in their lives. Since the concept of control was so central to the testimony of almost every patient, it will now be discussed in some detail.

'Control'

Patients sought to fill their 'unhappiness gap' by the close and minute control of food. Almost all participants showed great self-awareness of this process. They explained that they were redressing a shortfall in areas of their lives where their needs remained unmet, by exercising control over food. Somehow this single activity enabled them to keep at bay the torrent of pain which threatened to overwhelm them and which they would otherwise have experienced over the negative events of their lives. Their self-starvation assuaged the sense of chaos to which earlier traumas had given rise. It was around this issue of control that some of the most illuminating testimony was gathered. John for example explained:

> control is the major part ... of anorexia, really it's em control ... if you put control and food together then that that brings you an eating disorder because they're the two big things ... the two words that associate me to anorexia is food and control.

John later suggested:

> the control sort of thing [is most important in anorexia] rather than my appearance. It's the buzz that I get ... the controlling ... the feeling that I'm good at something em and that I'm being tight, I'm being organised, I'm being precise, I know what's going to happen, I know that I'm having say this for dinner, this for tea ... Everything, it's ... like my life ... it's a book.

Other participants made a point of explaining that anorexia became a way of controlling things in their own lives when they felt they did not have control over anything else. When asked why it should be in the area of food that the patient should choose to exercise control, Christine explained, 'It's the one part of your life that you can control what you eat ... it's commonly the one thing in life that you can control and ... it's just sort of, well, a means of that control ... you know.'

Other respondents echoed Christine's opinion. Julie suggested that even if she couldn't control anything else, at least she could control food. She thus felt the major part of her illness was wanting to be in control much more than it was about wanting to lose weight. As she explained:

> I think em it's a way of gaining control over your life. If you don't feel in control over sort of like your feelings ... you have control over your food and it's something that … n-nobody can take away from you.

The overriding sensation experienced by patients was a sense of terror at the prospect of relinquishing this control. Were her stomach to distend after a meal, Gail explained

> I just think that… I'd be losing control, that I hadn't sort of kept something tight ... it's sort of that I've let something go ... I don't feel as skinny as I did and I don't like that feeling ... It feels dangerous to me. It makes me feel out of control.

By exercising control over food, respondents felt they were somehow offsetting potential disaster in other areas of their lives. Angharad explained that as she carried on losing weight it made her feel good. It gave her a focus, eventually becoming the overwhelming influence in her life 'as long as I could hang on to that, everything else was going to be all right – and that's why it's so difficult here [in the hospital] that aspect [is] taken away from you'.

This may explain why participants experienced anxiety over the treatment regime at the Eating Disorders Unit. As part of this regime, patients were required to eat three meals a day. Several participants believed that this would remove the only locus of control they had. They spoke of the anxiety they experienced at the prospect of eating so 'much'. Ann for example explained:

> you have the control – you've done something with your body nobody else could do – you've done it. That's ... really really hard – handing that control over ... watching your body grow and grow and you're thinking don't let it go too far, don't let it go too far.

Participants were therefore engaged in self-starvation as a strategy of control to offset the lack of control they experienced in other areas of their lives. Patients were proud of their ability to control their food. The degree of control they were able to exert (along with their resulting weight loss) was a source of considerable enjoyment. Patients explained that their ability to control their weight gave them a 'buzz'. Getting this buzz was very important, and the process by which it was obtained will now be discussed.

The 'Buzz'

Every patient in this study enjoyed losing weight. It gave them a 'buzz'. Weight loss is something which most people find difficult – but these women (and men) were good at it. As Angela remarked, 'once I started to lose weight I felt good about it so y'know I sort of continued it and I loved it.' This point was reiterated by patient after patient. Like the subject of control, the 'buzz' issue was initiated by the respondent and the information surrounding it was volunteered in an unsolicited fashion. John discussed at length the enjoyment derived from being good at losing weight. 'It's the buzz that I get ... the controlling ... the feeling that I'm good at something'. Emma concurred 'Yeah it gives me, it gave me a buzz ... I've got a flat stomach that gives me the buzz ... it gives me a buzz the whole time'. Like Emma, Angharad explained that when she lost weight it really pleased her. She then began to deliberately want to lose more and it felt really good to be in control. All of a sudden she thought, 'Hey, I'm onto a good thing here', a feeling echoed by Samantha. 'I used to get some perverse buzz out of not eating', Samantha explained, 'because it felt ... like it was challenging'. As Julie remarked, 'getting on the scales and seeing that you've lost weight give[s] you a buzz ... you feel better about yourself'.

This sense of enjoyment and control prompted patients into further food restriction. They were caught in a cycle of food refusal, enjoyment, and further food refusal. This anorexic 'spiral' was described by many patients, and thus warrants detailed discussion. The key aspects of this phenomenon will now be described.

'Spiral'

The excitement or 'buzz' many patients experienced led them into a dangerous cycle of restriction, buzz, and further restriction. Lucy explained that an unanticipated consequence of losing weight was the satisfaction she derived from this. From then on the reduction in the amount of food she allowed herself became stricter and stricter, and she derived a sense of achievement from going that little bit further:

> losing that bit of extra weight that's kind of got the same effect from doing another day without that piece of food – yesterday and the day before I needed that, but today I don't need it ... and ... that was the new level going on from there.

Many participants explained that the more they lost the more they wanted to lose. As Angela reported, the anorexia cycle just takes over, and regardless of how much weight one loses one wants to be less and less and less. In Emma's words, 'it kind of escalated a bit and I didn't realise how far it had gone'. Samantha concurred:

> the trouble was the goalposts kept shifting because em ... when I started restricting I started off with saying 600 or 700 calories a day but then that wasn't good enough that had to go down and it just kept going down and down and down until I wasn't eating much at all and trying to live when you're not eating – you just sort of, well you lose a grip of things – I didn't see that at the time – I thought I was coping.

'Obsession'

This ever increasing concern with stricter and stricter food refusal led many participants to equate their illness with an obsession. Obsessional behaviour describes a state of mind where a specific course of action, such as food refusal, must be followed (Beech, 1978). Failing to carry out this action is unthinkable since the anxiety thus produced is impossible to bear. Emma described the way she became obsessed purely with the amount of food she was putting into her stomach. She was terrified by how full she might get. 'I never wanted to be full ... I had to be absolutely starving hungry ... for when I went home so that I could eat ... something at home ... but whatever I ate ... it had to be the smallest amount I could possibly eat.'

The obsessional avoidance of food and mealtimes led patients to develop various ruses to put off the fateful moment when they might have to consume a meal. Ann, for example, explained that she had reached the stage where she simply could not be at home during meals. She would prepare cold food for her family, but would be unable to eat any of this food herself. To avoid mealtimes, she would study late in the library or stay behind at work.

The elaborate strategies through which patients managed to avoid food were discussed by several respondents. Lucy described the rituals she engaged in around food as 'fine tuning' of the control. She had to eat her tea off a certain plate, or use a certain knife to eat a certain food. Selecting this plate and knife, she would carefully arrange the cutlery on the table, elaborately tinkering with the food on the plate, just so she could put off the moment where she was going to have to sit down and eat. She recalled standing around waiting for the minutes on the clock to tick by because she allowed herself to eat only at certain times. It was important to her that a certain amount of time elapsed between meals because that gave her the best chance of passing the next few hours 'without flaking out'. She explained that she would move her day around so that things would happen in the way she wanted. Even at work she would always have a plan to suit emerging circumstances:

> I was quite good at it you know, er, like moving my day around ... I could [even] sort [work] out so that things would happen in the way I wanted them to rather than like be affected by other things and certainly if they were going to be affected by other things I would always have plan B ready to er like suit whatever circumstances I thought were coming up.

Gail also explained how she had 'a lot of rules in her head' concerning how much food and drink she was allowed. She would plan in her head weeks in advance to account for every eventuality. This obsessionalism extended into other areas of her life as well as food. She engaged in cleaning rituals, rituals of organising household objects, and was even obsessive about certain TV programs, becoming highly anxious if she missed her favourite soap. The primary focus of her obsession however was with what she ate. As another participant, Samantha, explained:

> The bad part is that every waking hour of the day and sometimes even the night you think about food. You ... constantly crave food em and you think of ways em where you can get out of eating it.

Others described themselves as obsessed with calories. Emma disclosed an obsession with fat, and could recount exactly how many grammes of fat were present in any food. Samantha described her tendency to draw up lists of forbidden foods and allowed foods. As her strategy of food refusal became stricter and stricter, her list of forbidden foods kept getting bigger and her list of allowed foods smaller and smaller. 'It was just a way of me punishing myself for things that I didn't feel adequate in.' As she managed to relinquish some of her obsessions, she 'grabbed hold of others', and her weight continued to drop off.

Several participants described how this obsessionalism would also manifest itself in their responses to other women, either friends, passers by, or women on billboards or on television. Emma explained that she would constantly compare herself with women she saw on TV, particularly in relation to the flatness of their stomachs. Ann would similarly compare herself to passers by in the street. This obsessional state was described as trance-like by several participants. Christine, for example, described herself as being in 'robot mode', where nothing anyone said had any effect on her – her only concern was her relentless pursuit of thinness.

'Perfectionism'

Many linked their obsessional ability to exercise control over food with perfectionist traits in their own personalities. Several explained that they set very high standards for themselves in all areas of their lives. Rachel remarked that she had always tried to be as perfect as she possibly could. She felt that she always had to do the very best. 'It became hard then if you didn't do something quite as well – it became a major catastrophe – not just "oh dear, try again".'

Emma also described herself as a perfectionist, suggesting that she 'had all these obsessions and things', that she had to do. This was reiterated by Gail who believed that 'the obsessional stuff has come in because the anorexia wasn't enough to sort of make me feel better.' John too explained that:

> I have a very high em standard that I've set myself and you know whatever I do I think I'm not good enough ... I think I ought to perfect a ... certain thing all the time and it ... really affects me [if] I thought ... I weren't being hard enough on myself ... I've got to be stricter.

Samantha similarly explained that she enjoyed not eating because it was challenging, proving that she could set herself goals and attain them. She described how if she lapsed and failed to meet her target, she would punish herself in some way. She would swim or exercise or would go and walk several miles to burn off the extra calories.

It is hardly surprising then that some (though not all) participants described themselves as perfectionists. This perfectionism was brought into play in steeling themselves to refuse food. Equally these patients were sometimes the children of similarly perfectionist parents. This was often a source of deep pain in their lives. Lucy for example, felt that her parents had very high standards, but were less practised at congratulating her when she had done well.

Others however described their parents as loving and supportive. Gail expressed considerable anxiety over the thought that anything should happen to her parents 'I don't know what I'd do really'. Paula also described herself as close to her Mum, and for Angela the trigger to her anorexia had been the grief she experienced after the death of a beloved father.

'Anorexia is not just slimming'

Patients gave a clear and intelligent account of the complex factors leading to their illness. As well as identifying what had caused their illness many patients were equally clear what had not. Almost all patients expressed anger and frustration at the implication that anorexia was simply a desire to be thin and look like the women they had seen on the television. In Lucy's view, a significantly more serious dysfunction lay behind anorexia than simply an obsession with fatness and dieting. Lucy was also irritated by the suggestion that anorexia was no more than 'slimming gone mad'. By emphasising the link between slimming and anorexia, doctors missed the point about what was actually causing the disorder. Such a one dimensional analysis was, Lucy felt, quite dangerous since it belittled the illness. To people with no understanding of the disorder such an analysis rendered the sufferer as little more than a silly girl who wanted to look like a model in a magazine:

> to think that people would actually really think that you would starve yourself to the point where you can barely stand up because you wanted to be a bit thinner and look like somebody who was on the television is quite insulting in a lot of ways ... I suppose ... by ... improving people's self-esteem, you know, by placing more importance on that, making them realise that they don't have to look like somebody on the telly ... that would break the connection between the two anyway.

Christine also felt that reducing anorexia to a desire to be thinner was absurd. Christine believed that, sadly, in many people's minds anorexia was simply a disorder exhibited by adolescent girls who want to be thin. This was a markedly inaccurate view of the disorder, in Christine's opinion, and one which made her angry. In Christine's view, and in the view of several other patients, anorexia was much more than a cosmetic strategy. The disorder was so complex that Christine herself could not really say she fully understood it even though she was going through it. What may start as a desire to lose weight soon metamorphosed into a focus for all kinds of unhappiness. If it was simply a diet that had got out of hand, anorexia would be an easy disorder to dismiss and still easier to treat. Anorexia, for Christine, was a disorder where all kinds of feelings and emotions and insecurities were involved, and where dieting was merely a conduit for an underlying welter of confusion, unhappiness and pain.

A Sociological Explanation for Study Findings on 'Fat Phobia'

Patients were clear therefore that anorexia was not merely about dieting and weight loss. In the current study many patients emphasised unhappiness and lack of meaning in their lives as being central to the development of their illness. They appeared to be more concerned with these issues than they were with weight loss per se. The rich narratives volunteered by these patients were difficult to incorporate using the mechanistic, bio-technical models applied to anorexia (APA, 1980, 1994). The closed ended criteria currently applied to the disorder, with their emphasis on fat phobia, show a poor fit with the real experience of what has caused anorexia as identified by patients in this study. The imposition of pre-existing medical categories may serve to marginalise patients' real of experience of anorexia nervosa. It is thus important to define the illness using deductions which are negotiated and shared between the patient and the doctor (Kleinman, 1988).

Anorexia 'exhibits a rapid illness evolution as the cultural symbols communicated by food and body shape change' (Lee, 1995, p.34). 'Different explanatory schemes "leap and glee" upon its baffling features at various times' (Lee, 1995:34). Perhaps more than any other illness then the form which anorexia nervosa takes is culturally and historically specific. The assumption that there is a single underlying problem which manifests in anorexia nervosa is highly questionable. Rather there is an on-going process of cultural change and re-interpretation in the rendering of anorexia in the form (or forms) which it takes today. This analysis of this 'multi-forme' anorexia (Lee, 1995:34) requires a patient centred approach, which incorporates the highly complex reasons for self-starvation described by patients in the current study.

Patients explained that anorexia was not principally about fat phobia. If patients rejected this key element of the clinical explanation, a further logical question was whether other elements of the clinical model were also rejected. Another symptom which clinicians identify as central to anorexia is 'fear of maturity'. Not one patient in the current study, however, reported this symptom. While some patients may have expressed trepidation about making decisions and taking responsibilities, no patient described this as a fear of maturity, and no one wanted to return to their childhood days. In fact some patients described a disruptive and dysfunctional childhood, which they would be unlikely to want to re-visit. This suggests that the 'fear of maturity' construct may not always be supported by data.[2] Nevertheless, this construct remains pivotal to the clinical model. It is therefore important to theorise why 'fear of maturity' remains so central. Using a feminist approach, I will now explain why this symptom continues to be offered as an explanation for anorexia.

2 In this respect findings from the interview data were consistent with findings from the questionnaire data reported on page 136.

A Feminist Explanation for Study Findings on 'Fear of maturity'

If so few patients experienced 'fear of maturity', it is appropriate to ask why this symptom has been identified as a cause of the disorder. I would explain this by referring to the different constructions of 'masculinity' and 'femininity' under patriarchy. Femininity under patriarchy is rendered in negative terms (Malson, 1992). The male is constructed as 'normal', against which femaleness is constructed as 'other' (Malson, 1992). Negative definitions of femininity have important implications for the construction of 'female' illnesses. The knowledge definition surrounding such illnesses has a profoundly sexist dimension and anorexics are thus depicted as appearance obsessed teenagers, fleeing from adulthood.

No patient in the current study described her illness as fear of maturity, but even if patients were retreating from adulthood, who could blame them? I agree with Orbach (1993) that those patients who do experience this symptom are engaging in a legitimate protest against the adult female role. For women, under patriarchy, a full realisation of selfhood is impossible since the socially constructed self to which people are taught to aspire, (while nominally sex-neutral), is in fact masculine. Using this analysis, the rejection by women of their 'inevitable' destiny as downgraded female adults seems entirely understandable.

A corollory of the fear of maturity symptom is the notion of the 'anorexogenic' mother. However, no patient specifically described failings on the part of her or his mother as germane to their illness. While three patients described cruelty and neglect on the part of their fathers, and a further one patient described general neglect by both parents, no-one cited their mother's behaviour in particular as a key contributor to their illness. That patients in the current sample made almost no mention of their mothers in this regard is very interesting indeed. Such a finding runs counter to prevailing psychiatric knowledge which identifies maternal neglect as central to anorexia. Whether such neglect centres on feeding practices in early infancy

(Crisp, 1995) or on a failure to instill self-sufficiency and independence in her anorexic child (Bruch, 1978), it is nevertheless repeatedly invoked as a cause of the illness.

It is therefore interesting that patients in the current study did not report an especially poor maternal relationship. There may be two reasons for this. Firstly, the current sample may simply have been unrepresentative in this regard, and among other anorexics, the mother's 'contribution' may be more fully discussed. However, there may be a second explanation. Mothers may be much less 'anorexogenic' than is sometimes suggested (Ruskay-Rabinor, 1994). If we accept this latter point, we need to explain why psychiatric knowledge continues to cite mothers as 'causing' the illness.

Sexism in psychiatry is well documented (Mackler, 1976, Ussher, 1991). Ussher (1991) and Hepworth (1999) have traced the processes by which psychiatry objectifies women. This is reflected in psychiatric aetilogy, where a group of women, mothers, are cited as the 'cause' of mental disorder (Caplan, 1990, Mackler, 1976, Grolnick and Gurland, 2002, Wedenoja, 1991, Ruskay-Rabinor, 1994, Ussher, 1991). In a society which expects mothers to shoulder the full weight of child care, disruptions in a child's development are viewed as failings on the part of the mother (Ruskay-Rabinor, 1994). The findings from the current study, however, question the usefulness of placing such a construct in a central position when accounting for anorexia.

According to the results of this study, mothers are not to blame for failing to prepare their daughters for adulthood. In psychiatry, however, fear of adulthood is viewed not just as a flight from maturity, but also as a flight from sexuality (Crisp, 1995). This symptom is also highly value laden. It contains the assumption that the sex role constructed for women is unproblematic, and that females should accept this role without question. When we examine this role however, it is evident that it is far from problematic for women. Women are expected to be constantly sexually available to men, regardless of their own inclination or preference. It is males, according to this model who should set the sexual agenda, an agenda to which women should conform. Women who assert their own preferences continue to be characterised as unwholesome, predatory and comic.

The caricature of the sexually voracious female has long been a staple of British comedy,[3] and the stereotype that this represents powerfully illustrates acceptable behaviour for women.

In recent decades however, some progress has arguably been made in women's sexual liberation and women may now be more prepared to assert their own sexual needs. Articles on the female orgasm and the importance of foreplay and clitoral stimulation feature regularly in popular magazines and the sale of products to enhance women's sexual fulfilment has risen sharply (Chalker, 2000). One hopes that women thus feel a more total ownership of their bodies, and are ready to set their own sexual agenda. If anorexia is a flight from sexuality then one might expect its incidence to decline in an era where women's liberation has secured more sexual choice and freedom. However the opposite has been observed, namely that anorexia is 'on the increase'. This begs the question of whether the illness has more complex origins than the 'flight from sexuality' symptom might suggest.

Also it is noteworthy that three of the current sample were men, and it is interesting to ponder how this symptom applies to them. Anorexia is never described as a 'flight from full masculine sexuality', since, (unlike its female equivalent), male sexuality is constructed as a highly positive identity, which men would be unlikely to retreat from. Instead therefore, the motivation ascribed to male anorexia is constructed in feminised terms. Male anorexics are theorised as having 'ambiguous' or homosexual gender orientation (Robinson and Holden, 1986, Gregurek, 1994), and it is suggested that this 'problematic' orientation has contributed to their anorexia. That male homosexuality might be a positive identity appears not to be considered. For both men and women anorexics, therefore, the 'fear of sexuality' dimension appears to be applied in equally value laden terms. However, no patients in the current study discussed their anorexia as fear of sexuality, but instead used far more focussed language, describing unhappiness, longing, and a need for control.

3 See for example, the 'gagging for it' spinster in the 1970s 'Dick Emery Show', and Linda in the 1990s BBC comedy 'Gimee, Gimee, Gimee'.

In presenting my findings I aim to have explicated some important principles in the construction of psychiatric 'knowledge'. Some anorexics may well fear maturity, but others, as the current book illustrates, do not. This begs the question of why selective interpretations of the experiences of some anorexics are used to construct knowledge in a specific way. Could it be that the form of knowledge construction thus allowed reflects the mores and prejudices of patriarchal society?

A feminist interpretation of my results would suggest that 'anorexic knowledge' may be 'gendered'. This has implications not only for 'knowledge' but also for the way doctors view anorexics in the doctor-patient interaction. Research suggests (Ehrenreich and English, 1989) that such interactions may be influenced by the sex of the participants, particularly for anorexia, where patients are female and psychiatrists are often male. The doctor-patient interaction has been most fully analysed by researchers from the field of chronic illness (Kleinman, 1988). An account of the application of chronic illness theory to study data will now therefore be offered.

Interpreting Study Data using Chronic Illness Theory

Anorexia as a chronic illness

Anorexia is a chronic illness. It is a long-term condition (Lawrence, 1995) which can persist for decades. In the current study, many patients had lived with anorexia for years. On first being diagnosed, several experienced a sense of shock (MacDonald, 1988). Ann, for example, rejected her diagnosis while Paula remained 'in denial' throughout thc course of her hospitalisation. The 'life course' of these patients was thus disrupted as a result of their illness (Bury, 2001:263). Emma, for example, reported that her education, financial situation and friendship circle had deteriorated, while John and Gail had lost all their 'non-anorexic' friends. These experiences of disruption, shock, isolation and poverty are, sociologists argue, characteristic of the life burden of chronic illness (Bury, 1982, 1988, Locker, 2003, Williams, 1984, Strauss et al, 1984, see Chapter 2).

Chronic illnesses may also carry a certain stigma (Goffman, 1963, Kleinman, 1988, Scambler, 2003b). Anorexia may be labelled as macabre and puzzling, which may force the anorexic, like the AIDs or the herpes patient, to hide her condition from others. In the current study, Ann, Gail, Ilsa and Barbara concealed their anorexia by wearing baggy clothes, and by fasting at work so that they could eat something at home. They were clearly afraid of being unmasked and, in Goffman's terms, 'discredited' (1963:3). In labelling people as chronically ill, doctors therefore wield considerable power.

As well as labelling people, doctors also label diseases. As indicated in Chapter 1, disease classifications are negotiated by the clinical community over a period of decades or even centuries. I have argued that doctors classify diseases according to the biomedical model, but such a model may not always be suitable for a chronic disorder such as anorexia. The limitations inherent in adopting a purely biomedical approach to the assessment of anorexia will now be discussed.

Limitations of a purely bio-medical approach to anorexia

Sociologists working in the field of chronic illness have explained that a purely bio-medical approach is inadequate for dealing with long term disorders (Bury, 1982, Locker, 2003, Williams, 1984). Such an approach is better suited to acute illnesses requiring 'magic bullet' cures (Kleinman, 1988). Anorexia however is a long term illness and may be better managed by listening to the sufferer's own interpretation of her disorder, and providing her with support in the daily management of the disease. By listening to patients and supporting them, clinicians will 'enfranchise' patients, giving them confidence to apply their own understanding to the interpretation of their illness. Rather than conveying to the patient that her knowledge does not count, the clinician thus honours the patient's perspective and places her at the centre of her own recovery.

When clinicians deal with chronic patients they may find the patients' personal stories messy and difficult to manage (Kleinman, 1988). It is easier to stick to organised, pre-specified interpretations than it is to really engage with the patient and work with her as an equal partner in her care. By allowing patients to find explanations that 'work' however, clinicians can enable patients to place their illness in the context of their lives, thus making sense of their disorders. Such an approach acknowledges that patients as well as doctors have important insights to contribute. By combining their knowledge, doctors and patients can work together to provide care.

As indicated in the current chapter, patients may have explanations for the origins of their illness, which do not fit neatly with existing medical models. Sociologists writing in the field of chronic illness have explained that doctors and lay people often have different explanations for disease (Bury, 1982, Locker, 2003, Kleinman,1988). It is common for a doctor, for example, to focus on the physiological deterioration of a specific organ, while lay people often have a more generalised view of illness, which incorporates its context and effects (such as having to take time off work). Patients may also describe different reasons than doctors for their disorder. They may for example attribute their illness to a serious life event (such as bereavement), rather than to classic psychological constructs (such as 'fear of maturity').

There is therefore a potential opposition between 'lay' and 'bio-medical' explanatory models of illness. As a result of this opposition, psychiatric diagnoses are not necessarily fixed but are arrived at in a process of negotiation (Williams, 1984, Lupton, 1996b) between doctor and patient. Helman (2000) and Fabrega (1974), identified two distinct paradigms in the process of illness negotiation. The first may be described as the 'scientific' or bio-medical model of illness. This model is held by the doctor and is based on 'objective' pre-validated assessments and the application of established diagnostic rules. The second explanatory model is the 'folk' or lay model. This model is held by the patient and encapsulates the common sense, everyday beliefs that patients hold about their illnesses prior to coming to therapy. The distinction between medical and lay models and the way in which these models combine in the process of illness negotiation, is central to the study of anorexia.

Bio-medical models are based on the results of clinical research. The task of medical research is to seek agreement among clinicians concerning what causes an illness. Once a consensus has been reached, it is possible to develop a scientific explanatory model for the syndrome. Such a model by reference to its basis in external scientific 'fact', may become very powerfully established, and may function to exclude other models outside its terms of reference. As a result, clinical knowledge about anorexia tends to take a highly specific form. Consistent with positivist science doctors tend to construct illnesses in terms of certainties. With each new study, new 'certainties' are uncovered, which then become established as incontrovertible scientific 'truth'. The study of the contingent nature of these 'certainties' and the social process by which they are constructed appears to feature little in psychiatric research.

The 'interplay' of lay and bio-medical models

In the patient/doctor consultation lay models and bio-medical models interact. While some power may reside with patients (in that they may challenge the doctor, or ask for second opinion), most power rests with the clinician. Also, for illness such as anorexia, the patient is almost always female and the doctor is frequently male. There is therefore often a gender dimension to the manner in which the illness is appraised. Several authors have noted the gendered nature of doctor patient interactions (Ehrenreich and English, 1989, Ussher, 1991) and have described the disenfranchising effects of the paternalism that may characterise such encounters. The authority of the (usually male) doctor may therefore enable him to suggest a particular (often gendered) model of anorexia.

The power invested in the doctor thus allows him to communicate a specific model to the patient. It is precisely the extent to which such models are communicated (and at risk groups predefined), that is a central issue in this book. The data presented in this study has attempted to identify that patients have their own very distinct understandings of what has led to their anorexia, but these understandings are often subsumed under bio-medicine's requirement that the patient should view her (or his) disorder in specific ways.

> Doctors presume that their professional belief systems are 'objective'. Often ignorant of social theory which suggests that social actors actively negotiate and construct their own reality, doctors may trivialise lay beliefs and relegate the patients' own accounts to a subordinate position in the search for explanatory models. If eating disorders are to be located in their wider social context then the role of the professional in negotiating and determining illness behaviour must be examined. The symbols and manifestations of illness are influenced and constructed by a range of phenomena, including the 'constraints of a given medical theory'. (Swartz, 1987:617)

Frequently, this theory is encapsulated in the application of closed-ended rating instruments to the investigation of anorexia nervosa. The Eating Disorders Inventory, (Garner et al, 1983b), the Eating Attitudes Test, (Garner and Garfinkel, 1979), and the Eating Symptoms Inventory (Whitaker et al, 1989) have all been applied to the assessment of anorexic symptoms. Such rating tools may often serve to disenfranchise the patient's account by privileging certain areas of enquiry while excluding others. There is therefore an argument for the introduction of a much more flexible exchange in making an assessment of the causes of anorexia nervosa. In this way the 'lay understanding' of each sufferer will be respected.

Conclusion

At the end of the chapter what do the findings from the open-ended data tell us about the central research question tested by this study, namely that clinical 'knowledge' about anorexia may not always reflect patient's experience? Clinical 'knowledge' largely tends to construct anorexia as comprising intense fear of fatness. The open-ended data gathered in the current study suggest that anorexia is not chiefly about fear of fatness, and for this dimension the clinical model did not appear to apply to the current sample. Similarly, patients did not report 'fear of maturity' and in this regard patient's testimonies raise problems with the validity of the narrow clinical model. Such a model may not fully encompass the diversity of patient's experience as described by patients in this study.

However, this scientific model informs clinical constructions of anorexia. Such a model may ignore lay accounts in favour of medical ones. The difference between lay and medical interpretations has been widely discussed in the current chapter, particularly with reference to research from the field of chronic illness. I argued that clinicians may find chronic illnesses (such as anorexia) 'untidy', and may thus seek to find ways to 'compartmentalise' them. This may lead doctors to 'sidestep' patient accounts in favour of their own medical constructs. Such a process may be further exacerbated when (as in the case of anorexia) the patient is usually female and the doctor is often male. This gender difference may further aggravate the difference in power between the patient and the doctor. By adopting a model which honours patients' accounts, however, both male and female doctors can empower patients and enable sufferers to contribute to their own recovery.

In the current study, patients' own accounts, though rich and varied did incorporate some aspects of the clinical model. For some clinical dimensions such as 'control', 'obsessionalism' and 'perfectionism', patient transcripts concurred with, rather than diverged from, the clinical model. This may suggest that such dimensions, rather than being misleading stereotypes, are in fact helpful and accurate in theorising anorexia. According to the results gathered by the current study, it appears that patients do use anorexia as a strategy of control to offset a sense of a lack of control in other areas of their lives. Many patients also describe themselves as obsessional and perfectionist.

A key finding from the current investigation was therefore that patients do use anorexia as a strategy of control. However, even in relation to this dimension we should sound a note of caution in presenting the study's results. Patients were actors in a clinical environment. Some participants, as a result of their experience in hospital may have begun to construct their illness using the medical discourse of psychotherapy. Concepts deployed by psychotherapists in describing anorexia may have been acquired by patients and used by them to account for their disorder. The next chapter assesses the extent to which respondents appear to adopt the vocabulary of the psychotherapist when describing their anorexia.[4]

4 Excerpts from Chapter 7 also appear in Dignon, A., Beardsmore, A., Spain, S., and Kuan, A. (2006), 'Why I won't eat: patient testimony from 15 anorexics concerning the causes of their disorder', *Journal of Health Psychology*, 11,6,942–56.

Chapter 8
'I've spent a lot of time in hospitals': The 'Medicalisation' of Anorexia

This chapter consists of two distinct sections. In the first section, the words which patients use to describe their illness are presented, and the extent to which these words consist of medical terminology is considered. The second section examines the dialogue between the doctor and the patient (and assesses whether this dialogue is also 'clinicalised'). The two sections therefore focus on different aspects of the interviews to describe the 'medicalisation' of anorexia. The first of these sections, examining the words patients use, will now be presented.

'Medicalisation' in the words patients use

In this part of the chapter patient testimony is examined to establish whether patients describe their disorder using clinical jargon. The section will examine the extent to which patient accounts are informed by the psychiatric approach. In presenting this analysis, it is important to note that patients were actors in a clinical environment. They were being interviewed by a doctor, and it is feasible that, because a doctor was asking them questions, they may have made a special effort to answer using clinical terms. Their descriptions of their disorder might thus have been different had they not been talking to a clinician.

Some participants showed great awareness of these processes and suggested they may have described their disorder differently in a non-clinical environment. Anorexia is a chronic disorder and there are periods when it is in remission. Some patients explained that during these periods, they viewed anorexia in a less medicalised way. The flow of their conversation, however, and the spontaneity and fluency with which they used clinical vocabulary, suggested that they used this vocabulary automatically, and that it had become for them a natural and 'common sense' way of describing their disorder. The manner in which patients talked about their anorexia was captured by coding the transcripts into specific themes. This coding process will now be described.

Coding the data

Through the use of thematic analysis (Hewitt-Taylor, 2001) a core category 'Anorexia is medical' was produced. This category encompassed the process by which patients viewed their anorexia in medical terms. The category 'anorexia is medical' could be considered as a universal category as it encompassed all other categories. Five sub-categories were also identified:

'Deeper psychological issues lie behind the disorder'
'I've spent a lot of time in hospitals'
'Control'
'It gives you attention when you're ill'
'Depression comes into it'

These categories are illustrated in the following diagram:

Figure 8.1: Constructing Anorexia as a Medical Phenomenon

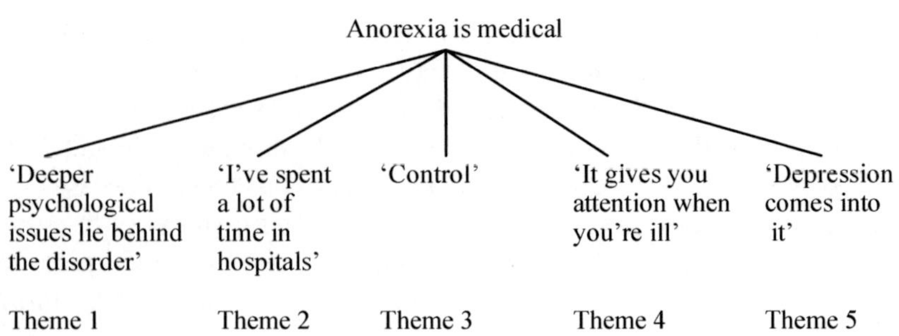

The coding process therefore identified five themes, numbered 1 to 5, which captured a significant and powerful dimension in relation to the manner in which patients medicalised their anorexia. Each of these themes will now be discussed.

'Deeper issues lie behind the disorder': psychologising anorexia

Psychiatric discourse surrounding anorexia has permeated popular culture to such an extent that even relatively 'uninformed' people now discuss the disorder in 'psychiatric' terms. Articles in popular magazines like *Bella* and *Best* describe anorexia as a quest for 'self-esteem', and television documentaries frequently identify the link between eating disorders and depression. Anorexics who wish to educate themselves about their illness now find a wealth of accessible resources at their disposal.

As patients in a clinical community, anorexics are stakeholders in the therapy they receive. Most are in hospital because they want to get well, and have a vested interest in the manner in which their carers model their disorder. It would be surprising if the constructions placed on the disorder by their therapists did not influence the patients' accounts of their health. Indeed, one of the key aims of therapy is to persuade the patient to structure her (or his) disorder in the same way as the therapist, as this construction is deemed to be a helpful, positive and therapeutic way of looking at things (Lawrence, 1998:97, Orbach, 1993:101). One might therefore expect that patients would be very likely to describe their disorder using the vocabulary of psychotherapy, and in the present study this is precisely what was observed.

Patients frequently used the term low 'self-esteem' to describe their feelings of unworthiness and pain. The phrase is widely used in psychiatry. For example Palmer (1989:41) states 'appearance and body size and shape are issues which may be of considerable importance, particularly to young women, in determining the individual's degree of self-esteem.' The phrase 'low self-esteem' was uttered by several participants (n = 12) in the current study and was used far more frequently than similar terms such as 'sadness' (uttered by no patients), or 'worthlessness' (uttered by 1 patient). In Hilde

Bruch's *The Golden Cage*, anorexics' testimonies are presented (Bruch, 1979:18–19, 74–5, 86, 135–9). The phrase 'low self-esteem' does not appear in any of these excerpts, nor is it used in Bruch's commentary on the transcripts she presents. It may be considered therefore to be a term that has been coined comparatively recently (Palmer, 1989, Lawrence, 1998, Orbach, 1993). Clearly patients have adopted this phrase because they have found it useful in constructing their account of their own experience of anorexia.

Patients also used the term 'coping mechanism' to describe the function which their disorder fulfilled in their daily lives. Emma, for example, explained that she used anorexia as 'a way of coping', while Angharad suggested her disorder was 'a coping mechanism for me'. Samantha also suggested 'it was more of a coping mechanism'. Although the term was frequently used by patients in the current sample (and also by the interviewing doctor), it is absent from earlier analyses of transcripts of anorexic interviews (Bruch, 1979). The term 'coping mechanism' gained currency round about 1980, and has since been frequently used in psychiatric texts (Weston et al, 1998). It is not unreasonable to assume that patients in the Eating Disorders Unit have acquired this term and adapted it in their own account of their disorder.

Several patients (n = 5) used the phrase 'obsessive' to describe their illness. Emma explained that she had had 'various obsessions and compulsions about food for years', while Samantha suggested that the difference between herself and the average dieter was that her diet seemed to have 'become more [of] an obsession'. One patient, Gail, even used the abbreviation 'OCD' (Obsessive Compulsive Disorder) to describe the problems she was experiencing. The term OCD was 'slipped into' the conversation in a knowing way and one which indicated a shared understanding between herself and the interviewing psychiatrist.

Four patients (Richard, Lucy, Rachel and John) indicated that they had read around the disorder and had come to a conclusion about its origins based on their reading. When asked by the interviewer whether she understood the term obsessive compulsive disorder, Lucy replied that she had 'read something about it' and had consequently considered it as a potential cause of her anorexia.

'Entanglement'

Another concept applied by patients to the analysis of their disorder was the idea of 'entanglement'. His illness, Richard suggested, had developed as a result of emotional difficulties becoming layered 'one on top of the other':

> Over the ... last 19 years a lot of different factors ... have gotten interwoven and laid one on top of the other … an awful lot of things that have got layered one on top of the other make it a very complicated picture.

Similarly Gail reported that 'it all gets ... sort of intermingled', while Samantha suggested 'feelings somehow got all mixed up with food'. Three further patients actually used the word 'entangled'. Moira explained that weight and emotion 'got so entangled', while Richard suggested that 'image does ... get entangled'. Another patient, Emma, described how concerns over self-esteem in other areas of her life had become 'entangled' with issues surrounding weight control:

> if things start to go wrong in your life ... you begin to somehow think ... if I lose a couple more pounds then I'll be better at this, and weight somehow became entangled with all those feelings, and I thought that if I lose a few more pounds I'd become a better person.

Clearly 'entanglement' is an elegant and useful concept for understanding anorexia. It brings the complex entity of 'anorexia' under some control by allowing us to compartmentalise our understanding of it. At the same time it illuminates the illness and says something very perceptive about its origins. It would be remarkable if such a handy concept had originated in the minds of the patients alone, and indeed it did not.

In 1989, Palmer published a book called *Anorexia Nervosa: A guide for sufferers and their families*. The third chapter of this book contains a section entitled 'Entanglement', from which the following passage is taken:

> It may be useful to consider that anorexia nervosa involves the gross and inappropriate entanglement of two issues: on the one hand, weight and eating

> control, and on the other, what might be described as personal and emotional control. (1989:41)

It may be coincidental that patients in the EDU describe the same precursor to anorexia as that identified by Dr. Palmer. It is highly unlikely however that the label 'entanglement' would be used except in a 'received' context. Patients were therefore actively involved in researching and reflecting on their disorder and in analysing it as part of their therapy. They consciously constructed their illness in part by using the analytical vocabulary of psychotherapy.

'The anorexic cycle'

Anorexic textbooks frequently refer to the concept of the anorexic cycle. This describes a cycle in which patients initiate weight loss, experience satisfaction, and subsequently become locked in a pattern of increased weight loss, further enjoyment, and further restriction of food (Lawrence, 1998, Orbach, 1993). Bruch for example suggests:

> the first loss of weight may be accidental. [...The anorexic] may receive praise and admiration for this, take excessive pride in looking slimmer, enjoy it, and then decide to lose more weight to earn even more respect. (Bruch, 1979:61)

Seven patients in the current study described themselves as subject to this cycle. As Angela explained, 'the anorexia cycle takes over', while Angharad reported being 'caught in the cycle of anorexia'. It is interesting that patients should display a detailed knowledge of 'buzz words' for describing their experiences. It is not unreasonable to suggest that in order to acquire this knowledge they may have conducted research into their own illness. It is equally reasonable to suggest that where such research has taken place, the ideas thus acquired might influence the way the disorder is described. More importantly, such activity may influence not only the patients' descriptions of their disorder, but to some extent their experience of it also. By internally rendering her experiences using the constructs of psychiatry the patient is helping to 'create' her own illness according to the dominant paradigm applied to its analysis.

It appears therefore that patients were actively engaged in analysing their own disorder. They thus may have viewed themselves as partners with their carers in conducting their own therapy, and this may have given them considerable motivation to assimilate and apply a psychiatric model to their illness. Some patients acknowledged that the process of assimilating psychiatric constructs was influenced by spending time in therapy, and it is to a discussion of this issue that I now turn.

'I've spent a lot of time in hospitals': Definitions of anorexia are influenced by therapy

Patients were aware of their tendency to see their disorder in a specific way as a result of being admitted to hospital. Ann, for example explained that she called herself an anorexic because she had asked the doctor what her disorder was. When asked why she had an eating disorder she could not give an answer:

> it was very hard to say ... that I'm an anorexic ... I had to ask the doctor really. But you know as to why I don't know and I don't think you can give an answer why. I don't think there is an answer. Em – you are because you're here.

On being asked what the connection was between having traumatic experiences and deciding not to eat, Lorna, replied 'I can't connect it at all really but that's what the doctors say, you know'. Christine had also been unaware that she was suffering from a clinically recognised illness, until she had consulted a doctor. 'I didn't realise', she remarked, 'that I was getting into an eating disorder but obviously I was'.

Some patients were aware that eating disorder had been defined as an illness as a result of relatively recent publicity it had received. As Samantha remarked:

> Em – I think it's been around for many years. It's probably like other illnesses. I mean so many years ago we hadn't heard of cancer so much – I think that people are just becoming more socially aware.

Other patients suggested that their thought processes were affected by the current clinical state of their anorexia. In response to an enquiry concerning her disorder Emma replied:

> now I'm in here things are different so it's difficult to ... think, you know, what I would have told you about if I was living a normal life outside here.

Similarly Lucy explained that she would have given more negative answers to the interviewer's questions 'like before I had an eating disorder, if you know what I mean'. The way she felt about things now she suggested, was more extreme when compared to the way she had felt before she had had anorexia. This revelation implied that the phenomenon of interest (anorexia) was being manifest in an intense form, and this was being captured by the study. The manner in which the current study was able to capture this experience was further illustrated in Julie's testimony. Though still in the acute phase of her illness, Julie was beginning to enter the recovery phase. She thus explained that she would have affirmed many of the interviewer's questions 'two years ago but … I don't feel that strongly now'. When she initially received therapy however Julie would have been more likely to discuss anorexia in clinical terms.

'Control'

Patients were very aware of their propensity to construct anorexia in specific ways, as a result of receiving therapy. As we saw in Chapter 7, one of the key dimensions which patients applied to their accounts was the dimension of control. Therapists (e.g. Lawrence, 1998) frequently describe anorexia in such terms. Anorexics apply rigid control over food to compensate for a lack of control in other areas of their life. Most patients in the sample described this symptom. Richard however had initially rejected this analysis, and suggested 'control' was unimportant in the development of his anorexia. During therapy however he had changed his mind and had reached the conclusion that control was a key factor. When asked if he had always been conscious of the importance of control he replied:

> Never. No. It's – I've really come to ... recognise more in recent years, looking back at the last couple of years I've spent a lot of time in hospitals, and ... I've spent a lot of time looking at my problems and where the roots of it might be.

Christine also suggested that anorexia was about control. When asked whether she had come to this conclusion because 'other people had said [this] to you', she replied:

> Well I didn't believe it at first but as I've been going to therapy and talking to people it's become more apparent that it was a means of control.

Patients also believed that in presenting themselves for therapy, they were empowering professionals to control their illness. Ann, for example, described the sense of pride she derived from having sculptured her body into a super thin structure. She felt she had done something with her body that nobody else could do. Handing control to a professional to manage her meals was therefore terrifying. She described herself as vain, appalled at her decision to allow her body to grow. Permanently anxious, her overriding concern was to not 'let it go too far, don't let it go too far, but you've got to have faith in those around you'. Angharad also described her terror at allowing the nurses to control her intake of food 'that's what the staff are managing and it ... leaves you feeling really scared and vulnerable ... I use my eating disorder to cope and all of a sudden that coping mechanism's gone'.

'It gives you attention when you're ill'

The above discussion therefore suggests that doctors are invested with significant professional control. This empowers them to grant exemption from normal responsibilities to those defined as 'sick'. In this way, the infirm 'enter the sick role' (Parsons, 1951). The manner in which patients 'enter the sick role' has formed a central focus in sociology. The sick role describes a process by which the patient acquires a distinct social identity by virtue of being labelled as 'ill'. They usually take themselves to bed, and for the duration of their illness are excused normal social tasks. As Holton and Turner explain:

> the difference between feeling sick and being sick points to the existence of a definite set of social expectations for the incumbent of the sick role. There is the notion that a sick person is exempted from responsibility for their condition [and] has an obligation to get well [and co-operate] with the doctor's regimen. (1986:120)

Parsons' model of the sick role was the first to recognise that 'the social and emotional relationship between the doctor and the patient was an important aspect of the therapeutic process' (Holton and Turner, 1986:120).

Several patients in the present study were highly conscious of their psychological need to adopt the sick role. Rachel for example explained:

> When you're really, really thin you look ill and people don't put too much pressure on you – my mother and my mother-in-law and my family have always looked to me to be to be the strong one of the family em and as I get bigger and look fitter and better they all relax and they think 'Oh great, she's really looking better – now we can put the pressure back on' and inside I'm still, if you like, the anorexic struggling to come to terms with the body and the the thought of the pressure can frighten me to want to be anorexic again so that it's a ... continuous sort of battle that's going on.

When asked why people felt better about themselves when they were thin, Rachel suggested:

> Because we're vulnerable, because people can't put too much pressure on us. There's a safety, there's a ... security.

For Rachel, adopting the sick role was a way of coping. When she couldn't cope with everyday pressures, the illness would warn people that 'she can't take it, she's too thin ... you're hiding behind it until it goes too far'. This, Rachel implied, was a conscious process, a method of signalling to others that she was unable to meet the responsibilities of everyday life.

Gail also was frightened of the responsibilities which 'normality' might bring. If she attained a normal weight, she felt people would expect more from her. They would expect her to be doing a proper job, and they would think that everything was all right, when things were far from all right in her head.

> I suppose it's partly to do with looking ill. You know, if you're underweight then everybody knows there's something wrong whereas if you're normal weight then people assume that things are OK, when you can be feeling, still feeling far from OK.

Lorna enjoyed people commenting on her anorexia and telling her she did not look well, 'sort of being the attraction, you know er people taking notice of me I think'. John also enjoyed the attention which the sick role afforded:

> It gives ... you attention you know obviously everybody ... when you're thin everybody thinks you're ill. I'm really sort of frightened now I'm starting to get weight on again and yeah I still look thin but ... in a half a stone's time or whatever if I went totally good, people'd say 'Oh you look a lot better John' ... when you are ... really thin people look at you, and you get, you know, 'Are you all right?' sort of thing.

Patients were also aware of the extent to which being in hospital and mixing with other anorexics had helped to inform the way in which they viewed their disorder. Gail explained:

> the people I have met have all been people who've got problems themselves which again I feel more comfortable with [laughs] ... I find it much easier talking to people about how I'm feeling than I do having a proper, you know having a conversation with somebody because I'm more practised at talking about how I'm feeling than just having a general conversation.

At least one patient appeared to be developing the first stages of institutionalisation typically experienced by patients in 'total institutions' (Goffman, 1968). Gail for example explained that she had started losing weight at about the age of 13 and had 'been in and out of hospitals ever since'. Her entire adult experience had been in the context of being labelled as a patient. As a result she felt she had not had a normal adult life or normal relationships. She described how the first hospital she went to had an Adolescent Unit which housed a lot of people her own age. She ended up getting on really well with other patients, since every one of them had experienced the same kind of problem she had. Eventually she did not want to leave the hospital, since this would mean returning to school where she had been tormented and which she dreaded. She would be sent home for a weekend, where she wouldn't eat. She would thus lose weight and would have to stay in hospital for a bit longer, and 'it just carried on like that'.

'Depression comes into it': linking anorexia to other clinical phenomena

Some patients therefore recognised that the way in which they experienced their condition had been influenced by institutionalisation. Other patients identified a link between their eating disorder and other forms of mental and physical illness. Ann, for example, when asked about her anorexia, explained that 'depression comes into it', while Angela suggested that she had initially lost her appetite as a result of allergies and stomach pains. Having lost weight Angela felt good about it, and continued restricting her intake of food.

Angela's physiological illness contributed to her anorexia, but for other patients their anorexia had led to physiological illness. John, for example, explained that his weight loss had resulted in 'pancreatic failure', while Angharad suggested that her 'electrolytes got really out of balance'. It is noticeable that these remarks are couched in technical terms (such as 'electrolyte' and 'pancreatic'). An interest in such terms however was most clearly illustrated by Richard. Richard referred to 'zinc deficiency' and its relation to loss of appetite. He also discussed the link between fat and cardio-vascular disease, and believed that anorexia was a corruption of good ideas about healthy behaviour – such as minimising fat and taking a certain amount of exercise. Clearly, therefore, several patients described their anorexia in a physiological and bio-medical manner. Key findings with regard to this process will now be summarised.

Patients' use of bio-medical terms: a summary

Patients therefore appeared to have acquired a bio-medical model for describing their illness and referred to this model in the course of their interview. This model incorporated constructs such as obsessionalism, entanglement, depression and control. Patients found these concepts useful in describing their disorder but such concepts were developed in the first place by clinicians. Medicine places a specific construction on the activity of self-starvation, and this construction may thus be acquired by patients. It is important in this book to consider how patients may have come to acquire such a detailed clinical understanding of their illness. Doctors, largely for caring and therapeutic reasons, may educate patients to view their disorder in a 'medicalised' way. In the next section, the process by which the interviewing doctor 'steered' the patients into 'medicalising' their disorder is examined.

'Medicalisation' in the doctor/patient dialogue

In the previous sections, 'chunks' of patient testimony were examined to establish whether patients described their anorexia using medical terms. In the next part of the chapter, the dialogue between the doctor and the patient is examined. It was very important to focus on this dialogue. By appraising this interaction (as well as the patient's words) I was able to analyse the communication between the doctor and the patient, and to establish whether this contributed to the medicalisation of anorexia.

The interviewer in the 'anorexic stereotype' study was a practising physician. Even though she had agreed to take a social approach to the interaction (see page 74), she was nevertheless a doctor talking about an illness. It was anticipated therefore that she would 'construct' anorexia as primarily a medical, as opposed to a social phenomenon. This is exactly what was observed. Using extracts from patient transcripts, I explore the manner in which a clinical model of anorexia was communicated by the doctor to the patient. Initially, I examine the doctor's focus on physiological issues, such as weight, height and diagnosis. I then describe how the patient is steered towards viewing her (or his) disorder as a clinical illness with specific origins. Finally, I explore the application by the doctor of the construct of 'obsessionalism', often described by clinicians (Kaplan and Sadock, 1995) as central to extreme weight loss. Weight loss was frequently emphasised by the doctor, and a discussion of this physical issue is now presented.

'How much do you weigh?'

The patient was initially asked by the doctor about the causes of her illness. Some patients, however, tended to 'dry up' after talking on this subject for a few minutes. In these cases, the doctor filled the hiatus with physiological questions on weight and height. The doctor appeared to 'fall back on' such questions, because she felt comfortable in discussing these topics. They also appeared to keep the patient talking until she could be 'steered back' to discussing the 'causes' of her illness. In the session with Julie, for example, the following topics were raised:

> DOCTOR: How much did you weigh when when you were at your most unwell?
>
> JULIE: About 5 stone
>
> DOCTOR: And ... how tall are you?
>
> JULIE: 5 foot 3.

A similar dialogue occurred in Paula's session:

DOCTOR: Right – can I just ask how tall you are?

PAULA: 5 ft 4

DOCTOR: Mm – and what do you weigh at the moment?

PAULA: Five stone ten pounds I think.

During Samantha's session the following interchange took place:

DOCTOR: How old are you now?

SAMANTHA: Just gone 27

DOCTOR: Right – and how old were you when it all started?

SAMANTHA: Probably early teens

DOCTOR: Mm so what [weight] are you now?

SAMANTHA: Em hovering around 8 stone

DOCTOR: And how tall are you?

SAMANTHA: Five nine, five ten

This dialogue occurred in the very early part of the interview, and questions on height and weight[1] tended to be asked immediately after the initial question 'what would you say were the causes of your anorexia?' From the outset, therefore, most patients were encouraged to focus on the physical aspects of their disorder. Seventeen of the twenty-four patients in the sample were asked questions of this kind. Topics included height, 'target weight', age and disease onset. Matters such as the use of laxatives and gastric nasal tubes (for 'force feeding') were also discussed.

1 As explained in Chapter 3, I encouraged the doctor to ask such questions as she felt were necessary to maintain the flow of the interview.

'Do you think you've got an illness?': Persuading patients that they have a disease

Some patients, however, did not consider themselves to be ill. In these cases the doctor's clinical focus was even more apparent, as she encouraged patients to face the seriousness of their clinical condition. During the course of the open-ended interview, the doctor tended to 'steer' the patient towards conceptualising their disorder in clinical terms and accepting that they had an illness. The following extracts exemplify this process:

> DOCTOR: D'you know what your diagnosis is?
>
> PAULA: Em well I ... don't – and ... actually I don't think it is down to me. Sometimes I just wonder why I'm actually here.
>
> DOCTOR: Right – you're in the Eating Disorders Unit at the moment aren't you?
>
> PAULA: Yeah – Em … on Sunday I went in
>
> DOCTOR: Mm – and what do you weigh at the moment?
>
> PAULA: Five ... stone ten pounds I think
>
> DOCTOR: So … most people would say you were underweight. D'you think you are?
>
> PAULA: No
>
> DOCTOR: Right – so you … wouldn't actually say that you'd got an illness?
>
> PAULA: Hard to say. Sometimes I just wonder what people ... are making a fuss about
>
> DOCTOR: Mm – but do you limit what you eat?

The dialogue between the patient and the doctor continued, wherein the doctor guided the patient to consider her condition as an illness, and to reflect on its possible causes. A similar process was observed in the interview with Ilsa:

DOCTOR: Would you accept that you've got an illness?

ILSA: Yes

DOCTOR: Yes. I mean just looking at you ... you look underweight to me. How ... heavy are you?

ILSA: Er ... I'd gone up to 43.6 kilograms, [six and a half stone] when I was weighed on Sunday

DOCTOR: And how tall are you?

ILSA: About 5 foot 4, 5 foot 5

DOCTOR: So ... you would accept that you've had a problem?

ILSA: Yes, yes

In this dialogue Ilsa was twice prompted to accept that she had an illness ('would you accept', the doctor asked, 'that you've got an illness?', and later, 'you would accept that you've had a problem?'). In addition, the doctor remarked, 'I mean just looking at you ... you look underweight to me'. In this way Ilsa was persuaded to consider her experiences as clinically significant. Andrew also was persuaded to construct his disorder in clinical terms. Andrew conceded that he had an illness, but was reluctant to acknowledge that he was underweight. The following extract is taken from his interview:

DOCTOR: [Andrew] can I just ask you how tall you are?

ANDREW: I'm just under 5 foot 11

DOCTOR: And how much do you weigh?

ANDREW: 7 stone

DOCTOR: Right, so do you think you're underweight?

ANDREW: A little, but not a great deal

DOCTOR: So if you look at yourself in the mirror, what d'you think? D'you think you look thin?

ANDREW: Sometimes I do

Andrew clearly believed that he was not emaciated. His reply 'not a great deal' to the question 'do you think you're underweight' suggests he considered his behaviour to be normal. The doctor however challenged his reply ('so if you look at yourself in the mirror, what do you think?') which persuaded Andrew to concede that sometimes he did look thin.

The doctor sought the patients' agreement with a clinical interpretation of the disorder. This agreement was often forthcoming, but in some cases, (such as Paula's above), it was not. Paula thus received additional prompts to guide her towards a clinical construction of her illness. In Paula's case these prompts consisted of reminding the patient the she was 'in the Eating Disorders Unit', and that 'most people would say' she 'was underweight'.

Getting the patient to 'understand' how her/his problem has arisen

The doctor appeared to suggest that anorexia was caused by specific pre-cursors. These included the use of anorexia as a strategy of control. This theme emerged in several transcripts. It was particularly important in the testimony given by Lorna. Lorna described how she felt very out of control when her weight increased. On being asked how she felt when she gained weight, Lorna replied:

LORNA: Oh … it's dreadful I've ... been on the [weighing] machine ... quite a few times and putting on weight's awful [laughs].

DOCTOR: Why does it feel awful?

LORNA: Em I'm so fat and flabby and horrible and ugly – it's horrible … I still want to lose more

DOCTOR: Do you still feel you're fat now?

LORNA: Yes I am at the moment – I've been less than this and that's what I want to be [pause]

DOCTOR: Why d'you think that would make you better?

LORNA: Because I'd look better and my clothes would fit

DOCTOR: What size clothes do you wear?

LORNA: 10

DOCTOR: So size 10 is too big?

LORNA: Yes I want to be size 8

DOCTOR: Right – why d'you think you want to be size 8?

LORNA: Cos I know then that … I am quite slim if I can get into size 8

DOCTOR: What do you think makes you want to look so thin?

LORNA: Em cos I want to look nice

DOCTOR: Do you actually see yourself as being fat and plump then

LORNA: Yes

DOCTOR: Cos when I look at you I don't see someone who's fat

LORNA: Don't you?

DOCTOR: No

Lorna was therefore persuaded by the doctor to reflect on why gaining weight should upset her and why staying thin would make her happy. The patient's commitment to remaining a size 8 was thus problematised by the doctor ('why d'you think you want to be size 8?'), and the dialogue was terminated by the doctor assuring the patient that she was not fat. Patient ideation was also problematised in other interviews. In the interview with Ilsa the following interchange took place:

DOCTOR: So … you would accept that you've had a problem?

ILSA: Yes, yes

DOCTOR: So what would you put that down to?

ILSA: It's hard to say but when I sort of think back to basic problems that I have ... I feel guilty and greedy

DOCTOR: Where d'you think the fear of being greedy comes from – what's that about?

ILSA: I've always always since early teens had that – when I've thought back over time – trying to sort myself out I can remember incidents very, very clearly of my early teens of feeling big and overweight and feeling just very, very guilty and greedy for eating in front of other people – very self-concious

DOCTOR: Do you have any idea yourself where that self-conciousness came from?

ILSA: No – just that I was an awful lot bigger in my early teens and feeling big and fat and having trouble getting clothes at that time that were fashionable to fit larger teenagers – It's probably a little easier now

DOCTOR: Mm – but it seems to have gone on to be more than just a diet

ILSA: What do you mean?

DOCTOR: Em to have got to the stage where you acknowledged yourself that you were severely underweight – what do you think?

ILSA: I honestly don't know … it was more just wanting to do as much as I could at the lowest possible weight – the ... sense of achievement

DOCTOR: It sounds like you wanted to be able to prove to yourself that you could … control [things] has there been a stage ... when you felt your health was suffering because of it?

ILSA: Yeah I suppose more in recent years – things got really out of hand about seven years ago ... and I wasn't able to do the hiking I'd done in the past

DOCTOR: Why d'you think that happened – what d'you think made it spiral out of control do you think?

ILSA: That's what I said to you … I don't know, I don't know, I don't know

DOCTOR: D'you get a feeling of anxiety if you eat?

ILSA: Yes … I'm always compensating … everything ... when I'm working … is geared around having the one ... meal in the evening with Chris [my partner] to be able to show him that I'm eating in front of him

DOCTOR: So it's almost a compulsion really?

In this extract, the doctor initially focuses on eliciting Ilsa's reasons for her disorder. ('Where d'you think the fear of being greedy comes from?'). Subsequently, however, the doctor steers the patient towards considering more pathological nature of her condition ('but it seems to have gone on to be more than just a diet'). When Ilsa requests clarification, she is reminded that she herself had begun to view her behaviour as serious (it 'got to the stage where you acknowledged yourself that you were severely underweight – what do you think?'). In the next question the doctor prompts the patient to consider anorexia as strategy of control ('It sounds like you wanted to be able to prove to yourself that you could ... control [things]'). This need for control however was actually damaging Ilsa's health, by causing anorexia. In a further question the doctor asks 'what d'you think made it spiral out of control?', and subsequently persuades the patient that this resulted from 'anxiety if you eat'. The doctor's final question 'So it's almost a compulsion really?' underscores this process of constructing the patient's experience as a compulsive disorder.

Compulsions or 'obsessions' are frequently invoked by clinicians as explanations for anorexia (Kaplan and Sadock, 1995, Russell, 2000). The patient seeks to obsessively control eating in order to offset the anxiety she would otherwise experience. Since obsession is so central to anorexia, I identified the frequency with which the doctor discussed this symptom (table 8.1), and an example of some of the dialogue in which this discussion took place is now presented.

Table 8.1: Frequency with which Weight/Height, and Obsessionalism were discussed in the doctor/patient interview			
	Number of patients who discussed the topic	Number of cases where the topic was initiated by the doctor	Number of cases where the topic was initiated by the patient
Weight/Height	17	15	2
Obsessionalism	11	6	5

'What about the obsessive stuff?': The construction of anorexia as an obsessive-compulsive disorder

The interviewer frequently made reference to 'obsessive compulsive' behaviour. An obsession denotes a state of mind where a specific course of action (such as self-starvation) must be followed. To fail to perform this action would result in a paralysing state of anxiety. Many patients described their behaviour as obsessional. John for example explained, 'I'm not having me breakfast, I'll have this for tea. Everything … it's like my life ... it's a book. Also if I'm going out it's got to be arranged weeks in advance'. Gail, Emma, Lucy and Rachel also described themselves as obsessive.

While such a description was often volunteered in an unsolicited fashion, the interviewer's response was uniform. Invariably she replied by deploying established therapeutic techniques for treating obsessive compulsive behaviour. These techniques involved encouraging the patient to consider their obsessive action, and the reasons for it (Beech, 1978). Many patients were thus guided into reflecting on why they were obsessively concerned with losing weight. Several reasons were supplied. This transcript, from Gail's interview, encapsulates some of the reasons volunteered for obsessive behaviour:

> DOCTOR: What about the obsessive stuff? What kind of stuff does that involve?
>
> GAIL: Em some of it's wrapped up with the food but not in the way that ... normally anorexics are – It's more to do with I have a lot of rules in my head of how often I can have things and how many drinks I can have and you know I

sort of go planning in my head weeks ahead to try and account for every eventuality of what's gonna happen and – I've got cleaning rituals and sort of having to organise everything and having to watch certain TV programmes and feeling really guilty if I don't

DOCTOR: What sort of TV programmes?

GAIL: It's normally the soaps and things but if I start watching something then I've got to keep on ... watching it – I find it really hard to miss then an episode

DOCTOR: What would happen if you did miss it?

GAIL: I don't know I just think … that I'd be losing control, that I hadn't sort of kept something tight – em it's sort of that I've let something go and

DOCTOR: And is it the same with the other things, feeling that things will be out of control if you weren't to

GAIL: Yeah, yeah

DOCTOR: So if you ... weren't in control what would happen?

GAIL: Em that's what I don't know really, what I think would happen ... I suppose I'd just feel that I wouldn't be able to cope with all the things flying around in my head ... I was quite scared of death as well and I think sometimes I'm perhaps trying to hold off sort of people dying or me dying or although in some ways I'd prefer to just die now and have it over and done with – I don't like the thought of living and then dying at the end of it

DOCTOR: What ... people are you frightened of dying?

GAIL: Mainly my family really ... especially Mum and Dad cos I'm, although I don't live with them now cos they live in S___ and I've stayed in N___ since I've been on the wards but I talk to them on the phone every evening and em I'd find it very hard if they were to die. I don't know what I'd do really

DOCTOR: So you somehow feel as though the rituals help to stop that happening?

GAIL: Mmmm

DOCTOR: Do you think that's sensible?

GAIL: No [laughs] no

DOCTOR: So you know at some level that it isn't – you just can't help yourself?'

Having encouraged the patient to consider their reasons for limiting food, the interviewer followed through with a sub question which again reflected established psychotherapeutic technique. She asked the patient to consider what was driving her obsession and what calamity would occur if she failed to perform the obsessive task:

DOCTOR: What did you feel was happening if you did eat, that's what I'm getting at really you see. What would have been wrong if you did eat?

If, for example, the patient's greatest fear was that her parents would die, and her ritualistic behaviour was an attempt to keep at bay the possibility of this happening, the interviewer would ask the patient to consider how likely it was that by restricting her food she would achieve this end. Was there any possibility at all that by failing to eat at specific times, or with specific cutlery, disaster would be more likely to strike? Having persuaded the patients to consider their behaviour in these terms, most concurred that their actions were illogical, but at the same time few expressed any desire or ability to alter their behaviour. A similar approach was observed in the doctor's interview with Emma. On being told that Emma was obsessed with certain things, the doctor replied:

DOCTOR: [sympathetically] What sort of things?

EMMA: Em well ... OK, it started when I was obsessed with fat and that's how I lost all the weight ... to begin with and I was absolutely obsessed with with fat

DOCTOR: Were you cutting fat out of your diet?
EMMA: Yeah … I'd studied exactly how many grams of fat was in absolutely everything and em I mean I could still now if you had er a dinner in front of you I could work it out – tot up to like within 10 per cent what, how many grams of fat you were eating … but then ... I got obsessed with the just purely the amount of food … I was putting into my stomach. I … started getting obsessed with

how full I was and I never wanted to be full … I had to be absolutely starving hungry

DOCTOR: So what was driving your obsession. What would have happened if you hadn't done that?

EMMA: I just ... couldn't be confident

DOCTOR: What did you feel was happening if you did eat, that's what I'm getting at really you see. What would have been wrong if you did eat?

EMMA: I would have just just absolutely hated myself. I couldn't do it. I'd have em felt like I had a big stomach and er I just couldn't handle it.

DOCTOR: So if your stomach had got bigger what would that have meant? … What was the significance of having a big tummy? Was it just that you had to control the size of your tummy and it showed how good you were at controlling things

EMMA: Mmm

DOCTOR: Or was it about wanting to look a certain way? Might it just be that you don't even know yourself?

EMMA: I don't know, I don't know. I don't know, I mean … I'm still absolutely obsessed with having a flat stomach

DOCTOR: So if you don't have a flat stomach … what would it mean?

EMMA: If I personally don't?

DOCTOR: Yes, for you, yes

EMMA: Em, that just can't happen [laughs a little]

In this dialogue the interviewer appeared to subconsciously construct her assessment of the patient's behaviour in psychiatric and clinical terms. The doctor in this study was very empathic and compassionate and attempted to communicate to patients an interpretation of their behaviour that was therapeutic and positive way of looking at things. At the same time however, such a construction showed little understanding of the anorexic's 'folk' perspective of self-starvation. This 'folk' perspective views self-starvation as functional in that it staves off anxiety, and gives the anorexic an area of her life (her intake of food) over which she can exercise positive control (Lawrence, 1998). Little acceptance of this viewpoint was apparent in the interviewer's construction of the disorder, as such an approach forms no part of psychotherapeutic assessments of obsessive compulsive pathology.

The patient/doctor dialogue: a summary

The interviews with the patients were characterised by the doctor's emphasis on physiological issues such as height and weight, and by her tendency to persuade the patient that she or he had a clinical disease. This disorder, the doctor intimated, had arisen from a need for control, and was identified as 'obsessive-compulsive' in nature. This process was especially interesting in view of the patient's tendency also to describe her disorder in 'clinical' terms. It is appropriate to ask where patients may have acquired this clinical understanding.

The following extract is taken from the doctor's interview with Moira. Prior to this interview, Moira, like all patients in the study, had been asked to fill out a questionnaire:

> DOCTOR: What do you think of the questionnaire[2] you've been administered?
>
> MOIRA: Obviously from reading magazine articles and things on the subject I do know that it's ... sometimes you know very high achievers, perfectionists[3] ... so ... some of the questions don't really surprise me.
>
> DOCTOR: Right, OK – did you find it easy to fill in?
>
> MOIRA: Fairly – some of the ones about the emotions were bit more difficult ... I think I would have found it more difficult say six months ago – but we've been doing modules on the Day Programme about emotion regulation – so I've been able to pinpoint the fact that I do find it hard to know exactly what I'm

2 See Appendix.

3 The patient was referring to a single question on perfectionism in the adapted eating disorders inventory (see Appendix).

> feeling ... cos sometimes I just feel completely numb, so I didn't find some of the questions taxing but I was able to answer them
>
> DOCTOR: Do you think that a lot of people that get an eating disorder have had different circumstances?
>
> MOIRA: Probably ... family problems, maybe self-esteem problems. I mean I know from doing some of the modules on the Day Programme it's a lot to do with emotions – it's a lot to do with self-esteem – with confidence, with self worth

It appeared from Moira's testimony, that patients had acquired psychiatric understandings while on the Day Programme, a course offered to anorexics, wherein they are taught therapeutic skills, such as emotion management. On the Day Programme, patients complete exercises which enable them to view their disorder in specific terms, since by re-thinking their illness in this way, they are able to adopt a more therapeutic approach to it.

As Moira also indicates, we also learn about the disorder 'from reading magazine articles'. It seems that as a society we talk (and write) more about anorexia than we used to and we use psychiatric terms such as 'obsessiveness' and 'control' to describe it. There is compelling evidence in both popular and academic media that the use of such terms is increasing (Dignon, 2006). For example, newspaper databases indicate that anorexia is being more frequently discussed in newspapers and that terms such as 'control', 'obsessiveness', 'self-esteem' and 'coping' are increasingly used to describe the illness (Dignon, 2006). Similarly, academic databases suggest an increase in the use of such terms in academic media (Dignon, 2006). From the patient's perspective, one of the most important sources of such discourse may be found in self-help books (Buckroyd, 1996, Palmer, 1989, Lindsay, 2000, Levenkron, 2000, Costin, 1997). These books convey in lay terms helpful information about the signs and origins of anorexia and how the disorder should be managed. They describe anorexia as an obsessive strategy of control (Lindsay, 2000:43, 72–5, 168, 169, Levenkron, 2000: 41–9, 21, 25, 28, 51, 79, 80, Costin, 1997:5, 6, 7–8, 122) used by sufferers as a coping mechanism (Buckroyd, 1996:35–50). Clearly such texts use a specific kind of discourse to describe anorexia nervosa. Patients are educated in the use of this discourse (e.g. on the Day Programme) and may be persuaded to apply this discourse to describing their disorder.

The Illness/ Disease Dichotomy

The doctor therefore largely conceptualised anorexia in terms of what Helman (2000) calls 'disease'. Disease denotes the state of being ill, as 'objectively' diagnosed by the clinician (see Chapter 2). Doctors claim to make these diagnoses scientifically (Kutchins and Kirk, 1997), but the diagnostic process is nevertheless socially constructed (Kleinman, 1988, MacDonald, 1988, Strauss et al, 1984, Berg and Mol, 1998). Clear variations in medical judgement are evident (Kleinman, 1988, Strauss et al, 1984, Lupton, 1996b, Helman, 2000, Berg and Mol, 1998), and 'the biomedical model [...] is open to differing interpretations, even among healthcare professionals' (Lupton, 1996b:93). As Comaroff (1982:63) explains, the 'medical model of disease in our society [thus] implies a cogent ideology'.

This 'ideology' may be communicated to patients. Physicians may 'mould the patient's [model] to make it fit the medical model of disease' (Helman, 2000:86). In addition, patients themselves may want to acquire a clinical understanding of their disorder. Patients' lay models have thus become increasingly sophisticated (Lupton, 1996b: 93) in recent years. A complex mixture of components may now be used by patients to interpret their illness (Lupton, 1996b).

> Mass media, home doctor books, novels, medical advice columns in newspapers and magazines, health education material, personal experience of symptoms [...] discussion with others experiencing similar symptoms and contact with physicians (Lupton, 1996b:93)

may all contribute to the patient's common sense model.

Patients thus have a wealth of available resources from which they may acquire clinical knowledge. At the same time as patients have acquired more technical understanding, it is evident that doctors incorporate their own lay beliefs into medical theory. 'Scientific' knowledge is thus produced from:

> Relationships [...] between the researcher, the scientific community of which he is a member, the knowledge which the community shares, and the broader religious, social and political currents within which the community exists. The upshot of this has been that the once-vast chasm between science and other symbolic systems has appeared [...] almost to disappear. (Wright and Treacher, 1982:7–8)

Medicine thus incorporates knowledge from the wider community, and at the same time the wider community is acquiring more medical knowledge. However

> while members of the lay population of contemporary Western societies may be exposed to more sources of information about health and medical matters than previously, due largely to increased coverage by the mass media and the publication of popular books about health and illness, the treatment of illness still relies upon the interpretation as well as the possession of the appropriate knowledge. (Lupton, 1996b:109)

It is only clinicians who through training have the expertise to successfully interpret and apply this knowledge.

Clinicians claim to apply their knowledge objectively, for example in the self-help books that patients access. In reality, however, their practice is often influenced by subjective, political and non-scientific factors. Political decisions, for example, are made in respect of access to services. Griffiths (2001), explains that access to care is rationed, where political choices are made concerning who receives treatment. In this way 'a small group of elite actors ration services for others [...] people are turned away [...] made to pay at least part of the bill and told that desired treatments are not covered' (Light and Hughes, 2001:561–2). The status and deservabilty of such cases however is decided politically. In a period of increasing caseloads and straitened resources 'professionals [...] draw the boundaries of patient eligibility in ways that suit their interests' (Griffiths, 2001:679). The 'amount of care [is thus] rationed [...] while [...] access to care' is similarly restricted (Bourgeault et al, 2001:633).

The rationing process demonstrates that the practice of medicine is a highly politicised activity. Doctors nevertheless often present their practice as objective and scientific. The scientific perspective tends to exclude any discussion of the cultural context of ill health, and the meaning of illness in the life of the patient, by focusing more on the syndrome than on the patient herself. The scientific model is reproduced (in diluted form) in magazine articles and self help books (Levenkron, 2000), the overwhelming majority of which are written by clinicians. Patients access such texts and the models contained therein form part of their account of their disorder. The acquisition by the patient of complex medical discourse therefore is an extension of medical power. Patients are not only compliant in the consultation, they also extend this compliance by 'boning up' on medical wisdom in their spare time.

The Importance of Professional Control

By communicating its view of knowledge to the rest of society, medicine has the power to influence what people will think about specific illnesses. Foucault (1979) explains that with the growth of professions such as medicine, the control such professions exhibit has permeated through into the microelements of ordinary life. Few elements of daily existence remains untouched by such control. The taken for granted folk understandings which patients have of their illnesses are therefore suffused by this controlling professional discourse. As a result patients and doctors unconsciously 'collude to solve a problem' (Lupton, 1996b:111).

This collusion may be understood, in Annandale's words as a 'mode [...] of living [...] tied to the sub-politics of medicine' (1998:18). When 'medicine [is] defined in this way [it] employs a market strategy which profits from risk' (1998:18). Quoting Beck (1992), Annandale explains 'not only is the spiral of medical formation and decision-making twisted deeper and deeper into the

[…] reality of the risk society, but an insatiable appetite for medicine is produced' (Annandale, 1998:18). In other words, in a society which identifies risk, (by for example, highlighting economic and environmental hazards to health), patients are increasingly becoming consumers of clinical services. They are hence more likely to form a partnership with the doctor in the clinical consultation.
Silverman explains:

> the greater involvement of the patient in the consultation is both emancipatory and constraining. The mistake is to treat surveillance purely as a function of professionals treating patients as objects of the clinical gaze. Surveillance works no less efficiently when we are constituted as free subjects whose freedom includes the obligation to survey ourselves. (1987:225)

In acquiring technical understanding from doctors, self-help books and television documentaries, patients are engaged in self-surveillance. Self help groups and magazine articles therefore facilitate the extent to which professional control may be exhibited.
As Lupton explains:

> empirically based investigations have demonstrated the ways in which bodies become inscribed by dominant discourses [...] how relations of power are [...] reproduced in everyday activities as well as by[…]medical practices, and how medical and public health ideologies are incorporated into lay knowledge of health and illness. (1996b:104)

Patients at the Eating Disorders Unit were suffering from a serious and debilitating mental illness brought on by the pain and suffering in their lives. Psychiatry has frequently succeeded in producing models for understanding illness which are illuminating and therapeutic. Hence the constructions which psychiatrists place on mental disorder are usually developed with the best of intentions in mind. They often serve to liberate and enlighten the patient as well as informing the world at large about puzzling and complex phenomena. Nevertheless, these constructions are often presented as unassailable truths by people who support them. They are rarely seen as consciously constructed models which can often serve to obscure and disenfranchise alternative explanations. What is interesting about such paradigms is that they become powerfully established in the general consciousness. They become 'second nature' to the degree that people no longer realise they are using them. In the lives of patients this may not only influence their construction of their disorder, but by enabling them to form a specific view of their disease, it will influence their experience of it also. There is a danger then that we may be thus influenced to such a degree by psychiatry, that the psychiatric model and this model alone, will limit our understanding of a highly complex psychological and social disorder.

Chapter 9
Conclusion

Introduction

In this book, I have discussed the manner in which patients become 'schooled' in describing their disorder using a certain model. This model was based on 'obsessionalism' and 'control', constructs which patients felt were important in causing their anorexia. I have also discussed constructs which patients did not consider important in causing their illness but which are nevertheless privileged in the clinical model. These constructs were 'fear of maturity' and 'fear of fatness'. This concluding chapter will summarise the study's findings particularly in relation to these constructs. The chapter will argue that fear of maturity and fear of fatness, while central to the clinical model, were unsubstantiated by data in this study. It will also explain that other elements of the clinical stereotype, particularly in relation to class and education, were also unsubstantiated by study data.

Synopsis of the Book's Findings

The findings of the book can be summarised by presenting a brief review of each chapter. In Chapter 1, a study outline was presented. The chapter argued that knowledge about self-starvation has taken different forms in different periods in history. Present day opinion on anorexia has evolved over a period of decades and is therefore a social product, as well as a reflection of external phenomenon. Anorexia was further discussed in Chapter 2, where a literature review of eating and anorexia was presented. The chapter described sociological research, particularly research from the sociology of chronic illness. This was followed by Chapter 3, which described the study methodology and emphasised the different types of data (open and close ended) which the study collected.

In Chapter 4 the nature of the psychiatric model of anorexia was described. Such a model reflected a stereotype of anorexia. The family (and its individual members) were identified as the 'cause' of the disorder (Bruch, 1978, Minuchin, 1991, Minuchin et al, 1978, Crisp, 1995). According to this view, the anorexic's mother has failed to prepare her daughter for adulthood, and has engendered in her a horror of growing up (Crisp, 1995). The anorexic is therefore unsuccessful in fully adjusting to adult femininity (Crisp, 1995).

Such a perspective, the book argues, views anorexia entirely at the level of the individual and fails to theorise socially constructed femininity as a potentially problematic identity. Little account has been taken by psychiatrists of the social context in which anorexia occurs. Some psychiatrists have however acknowledged the importance of society in the development of anorexia. These physicians, (known as socio-culturalists), have studied data on the age, class, education and residence of the typical anorexic. They have identified the 'stereotypical' anorexic as a young, bright, affluent city dweller (Bruch, 1978, Crisp et al, 1976, Azuma and Henmi, 1982, Hamburg and Herzog, 1985).

While acknowledging the importance of society, socio-cultural psychiatrists have failed to conduct a rigourous appraisal of the manner in which social identities (particularly femininity) are constructed. As a result, psychiatric theories have largely omitted any discussion of gender, and it has been left to feminist psychotherapists to address this omission in the psychiatric model. These feminists have placed the position of women and women's inequality at the centre of their analysis. Such a focus is essential when one considers the female 'demographic' of the illness.

Further demographic data were presented in Chapter 5. Information on age, class, education and place of residence was appraised to test the accuracy of demographic elements of the clinical stereotype. A key objective of Chapter 5 was to examine the accuracy of the stereotype of the bright, affluent, urban anorexic. By analysing data collected from anorexic patients (and comparing this with Census and Department of Education data), the value of the stereotype was appraised and prevailing myths surrounding anorexia were deconstructed. Statistics were presented to demonstrate that a similar proportion of working class to middle class women, high and low achievers, town and country dwellers, appeared in my anorexic group when compared to census data. I thus concluded that women from all social groups may and do experience anorexia.

I therefore suggested that the demographic stereotype is a social construction, generated by psychiatric researchers. Though some opposition to this model exists among 'mainstream' psychiatrists, this stereotype has remained in place for over 30 years. It persists because of its widespread acceptance by the clinical community. It is not only in relation to the demographic characteristics of the anorexic that a stereotype is evident, however. In relation to the anorexic's cognitive symptoms a stereotype may also be observed. In Chapters 6 to 10, the value of the cognitive stereotype was appraised. Chapter 6 presented information from a closed-ended questionnaire covering cognitive symptoms stereotypically associated with anorexia. The results indicated that the importance of 'stereotypical' symptoms (particularly 'weight phobia' and 'fear of maturity') in 'causing' anorexia was modest. However some symptoms identified by clinicians, especially the use of anorexia as strategy of control, were validated by the results from the closed- ended questionnaire.

The importance of control was further appraised in Chapter 7, where narrative data from the open-ended interviews was presented. Patient after patient explained that anorexia was about more than just dieting for cosmetic reasons to do with size. In view of this testimony, the book suggests that 'fear of fatness', so central to the clinical model of anorexia, may at best be a secondary explanation for the illness. In addition no patient described herself as afraid to grow up or as wishing to return to the security of childhood. This key element of the anorexic stereotype was therefore unsubstantiated by the qualitative data gathered in this book. There were however, a number of other symptoms, which did appear to be important in the development of the patient's anorexia. These included the symptoms of control and perfectionism, suggesting that these elements of the cognitive stereotype were genuinely reflected in patient experience.

Chapter 8 describes the 'medicalisation' of anorexia. The chapter explains that patients describe their illness using highly bio-medical terms, (such as 'obsessionalism'). Such concepts are sophisticated psychological constructs, developed in the first place by clinicians. Almost all patients however appeared to be highly versed in such psychological vocabulary. One forum through which this vocabulary may have been acquired is the doctor/patient interview. Detailed extracts of the dialogue between the doctor and the patient were therefore presented, to assess the process by which the doctor 'steers' the patient towards adopting a bio-medical view of her disorder.

Summary of the Study Findings

This study has therefore suggested that there are several areas of clinical knowledge surrounding anorexia that may be viewed as problematic. These areas are:

Age Social class Education Place of residence	Demographic dimensions
Fear of fatness Fear of maturity	Cognitive dimensions

The first theoretical perspective used in the book to interpret these findings was the feminist perspective, and a summary of feminist interpretation offered in the book will now be presented.

Summary of the Feminist Analysis Offered in the Book

Feminism places the location of women in society at the centre of its analysis of anorexia. By analysing the patriarchal nature of psychiatric knowledge, feminism can explain why the model of the diet obsessed youngster, afraid to grow up, persists. Such a model reflects the assumption that female adulthood is an unproblematic identity which women should simply accept. The unequal status, (both social and sexual) of adult women in patriarchal society is sidestepped in such a model. Fear of maturity also contains the assumption that the anorexic's mother has failed to properly prepare her daughter for adulthood. Such 'mother-blaming' in psychiatry is well documented (Caplan, 1990, Mackler, 1976, Grolnick and Gurland, 2002, Wedenoja, 1991, Ruskay-Rabinor, 1994, Ussher, 1991) and carries with it the sexist assumption that when something goes wrong in the life of the child, the mother is somehow at fault. Such a form of knowledge construction reflects the prevailing prejudices of patriarchal society.

No patient in the current sample described themselves as afraid of adulthood, and it is appropriate to ask why. 'Fear of maturity' is a highly value laden symptom which fits the model of the appearance-obsessed adolescent perfectly. It trivialises women's pain and detracts from the complex causes of an illness that is a deep-rooted expression of women's distress. In a field where aetiology is characterised by interpretation, it provides a 'plausible' model, but one which contains patriarchal assumptions and often fails to reflect patients' experiences. Little attempt is made in this model to appraise the problematic role of adult femininity.

As well as theorising 'fear of maturity', feminism may also be used to explicate the construct 'fear of fatness'. As Steiger (1993) explains the overwhelming preponderance of women in statistics for anorexia may not just be about the crude media inculcation of thinness as beauty. It may rather be the result of an institutionalised difference between men and women in obtaining opportunities for self-definition and self-empowerment. This difference between males and females is therefore less to do with media ideals and much more to do with the actualisation of selfhood. Instead of looking at the cosmetic issues, it might be appropriate to study the disorder as an exercise in addressing powerlessness. When we approach anorexia from this standpoint we may find that the illness can be effectively treated through the promotion of social and economic well being as well as the psychological health of women. Equal pay and employment status, adequate child care and maternity leave and protection from abuse, might all be seen as approaches to treatment from this perspective. In other words we will be unable to treat the effects of anorexia until we address the inequalities in the social world in which the anorexic resides.

In presenting my findings I hope to have explicated some important principles in the construction of psychiatric 'knowledge'. Some anorexics may well fear fatness, but others, as the current book illustrates, do not. This begs the question of why selective interpretations of the experiences of some anorexics are used to construct knowledge in a specific way. I have argued that this form of knowledge production reflects the mores and prejudices of patriarchal society. Because of this, I have conducted a feminist analysis of the results from the current study, and have used this perspective to analyse the clinical model of anorexia. This clinical model informs the manner in which the doctor discusses the patient's illness in the doctor/patient interaction. Such interaction may frequently be described as gendered, as anorexics are almost always female and the doctor is often male. This may exacerbate an already existing power imbalance deriving from the doctor's clincal authority. The body of research most widely applied to theorising differences in power between doctors and patients has been compiled by sociologists from the field of chronic illness, and a summary of the study's conclusions in relation to chronic illness research will now be offered.

Summary of the Analysis Offered based on Chronic Illness Research

Sociologists in the field of chronic illness have explained that doctors and patients often apply different 'explanatory models' (Kleinman, 1988, Bury, 1988, MacDonald, 1988, Anderson and Bury, 1988, Helman 2000:85, Freidson, 1970b, Fabrega, 1974, Fisher, 2001) to illness and disease. The doctor may have an elaborate explanatory system, negotiated by the clinical community over a period of decades, which s/he applies to the patient's illness. The patient however may view the illness much more in terms of the individual causes she ascribes to it, such as work stress or bereavement. She may also evaluate her disorder in relation to its impact on her life, such as its effects on her employment or educational opportunities.

Several commentators (Kleinman, 1988, Bury, 1988, MacDonald, 1988, Anderson and Bury, 1988, Freidson, 1970b, Nettleton, 1995, Helman, 2000, Fisher, 2001, Weitz, 2001) have described how the power vested in the doctor has secured for physicians the ultimate authority for defining clinical knowledge. These scholars have suggested that doctors have the power to define what constitutes illness. It is in the area of psychiatric illness that many of the clearest examples of the social construction of disease are to be found. Psychiatrists use their authority to select what they are interested in. They assume illness is an objective entity and use technical procedures to uncover it (Kleinman, 1988, Strauss et al, 1984, MacDonald, 1988, Nettleton, 1995, Kutchins and Kirk, 1997, Weitz, 2001). Thus, as many sociologists explain, psychiatrists bring a technical perspective to the illness consultation. This perspective is aimed at 'problem solving' through the use of 'technical control' (Mishler, 1984: 124). The patient's problems are therefore 'dissolved', (Mishler, 1984:126) into this system of technical-rational language. This technical perspective has been referred to as the 'voice of medicine' (Mishler, 1984: 95), or 'rational purposive action' (Habermas, 1970:105). This is contrasted with the lay perspective adopted by the patient, referred to as the 'voice of the lifeworld' (Mishler, 1984:95).

The doctor's technical-rational system (as reflected in the 'knowledge' discussed in this book) comprises what Thrift calls 'empirical knowledge'. This involves 'accepted procedures, accepted standards and assumes the correctness of existing knowledge', (1994:377). Empirical knowledge, Thrift explains, offers a 'rational explanation' and organises 'knowledge in a systematic fashion' (1994:375). It is acquired by an actor's membership of a specific social group, such as the clinical community.

It may also be argued that such knowledge and authority is embedded in and reflects patriarchal culture, where 'male dominance is interwoven with professional dominance' (Fisher, 2001:150). A sexist stereotype of anorexia is thus produced which constructs the sufferer as a recalcitrant female adolescent, with 'female' and 'adolescent' problems. These include fear of full sexual maturity and by implication fear of sex, contravening the male directive that women should display constant sexual receptiveness and availability.

This technical rational knowledge exerts a powerful influence regardless of the tenor of the doctor-patient consultation. In the current study the doctor was empathic and caring and dealt with the difficult issues raised by the patients in a therapeutic way. Doctors may not always be so supportive (Kleinman, 1988). Kleinman (1988) explains that the doctor patient relationship varies much more than one might imagine. Some doctors are patient-centred and empathic while others provide little emotional support (Kleinman, 1988, Strauss et al, 1984, Bury, 1988, MacDonald, 1988, Anderson and Bury, 1988, Berg and Mol, 1998). Clinical judgements may also differ hugely from one consultation to another (Kleinman, 1988, Strauss et al, 1984). Doctors may therefore view medicine and the clinical judgement it involves as an art as well as a science, but they nevertheless ultimately apply technical criteria backed up by medical authority.

Lee summarises this problem in apposite terms:

> medical diagnosis is a social participatory process, a creation of physician and patient together [...] bio-medically trained practitioners are obliged to filter [patients's] narratives through their familiar academic explanatory models and may be eager to see that their theories are consistently confirmed. In this

process of selective perception, they may often unknowingly exaggerate what is posited to be universal in [anorexia nervosa], at the expense of de-emphasizing the culturally particular. (Lee,1995:32)

This process of 'diagnostic stereotyping' (Lee, 1995:32) and 'theory derived professional interpretations' (Lee,1995:32), amounts to shoehorning complex accounts into the 'straightjacket' of prevailing psychiatric theory. Unlike in the case of organic disorders, it is difficult to validate diagnoses of mental illness using bio-chemical tests and procedures. There may therefore be considerable interpretation and subjectivity on the part of the therapist when making a diagnosis of anorexia nervosa. A temptation may exist to interpret patients' narratives so that they fit the established diagnostic criteria (APA, 1994,1980), and patients may be recorded as conforming to these criteria in circumstances where they may not actually do so.

A flexible approach should therefore be applied to the anorexic consultation. No longer should standardised rating tools limit the choice of questions asked and responses obtained. Equally the researcher's approach to assessing which socio-economic groups may be likely to contract the disorder should be open-minded, and the old stereotype of the anorexic as a middle class, urban, high achiever should be reconsidered. In this way the individuality of each sufferer will be respected and the importance of the socio-cultural context of disordered eating will be recognised. This type of approach would place as much value on the patient's accounts, as is currently placed on the functionality of existing symptom rating instruments. By setting the sufferer's illness in the context of her (or his) own account of its causes, the patient becomes an expert in her own disorder 'rather than having to colonize [her problems] into biochemically established norms' (Katzman and Lee, 1997:391).

Such a dynamic model would also help to incorporate the diversity in class distribution, education level and residential location observed in Chapter 5. The changes which may have occurred in the class and education of the anorexic population over the past few decades might therefore be accommodated. This model would also absorb the complexity of the personalised narratives (see Chapter 8) as well as the cultural contexts in which the events in these narratives occurred. As Banks (1992) explains 'The answer to the question about which aspects of culture are involved in anorexia depends therefore, on whether one takes the point of view of the bio-medical system or the varying points of view of the anorectics themselves' (1992:881). By developing a model of eating disorder etiology based on a complete picture of the disorder which views its manifestations and causes from both the patient's (emic) and the doctor's (etic) perspective, we can develop a picture of the illness, where no aspect of the patient's experience is overlooked.

Treatment

It is not within the remit of this book to discuss the treatment given to anorexic patients in any detail. Since the social context of anorexia and the socially defined nature of the illness will have implications for therapy, however, it is important to briefly discuss the therapeutic implications of viewing anorexia from a sociological perspective. By 'learning' the doctor's bio-technical model and reproducing this in her account of her illness (Chapter 8), the patient may arguably secure the doctor's approval. This may have significant implications for the level of rapport established and the resulting success of her therapy. The ethics of requiring a patient to absorb the clinical model in order to get well are however questionable. A willingness on the part of the clinician to listen to and accept the patient's perspective may have more positive implications for the treatment of anorexia. In Hsu et al's study (1992), patients reported that feeling understood was one of the key contributors to successful treatment.

Treatment which fails to accommodate the patient's perspective may be experienced as humiliating and ineffective. Behaviour modification, manifested in a contractual agreements whereby the patient agrees to be 'fattened up' is often experienced as a form of humiliating coercion. Some patients in the current study clearly indicated their unhappiness with such a regime (see Chapter 7), and several indicated that it failed to address the more deep-seated psychological issues that had led to their initial food refusal.

Psychiatric treatment often emphasises an adjustment model of health (Broverman et al 1972). The objective is to reconcile the anorexic with the reality of entering female adulthood, regardless of the problematic nature of such a role. In challenging the anorexic's fear of sexual maturity, therapy contains within it the assumption that the attainment of sexual availability is a key goal of psychiatric treatment. At the same time many psychotherapists attempt to persuade the anorexic to reconcile herself with often quite abusive families. Thus the treatment of anorexia is often a conservative and culture bound process. A less reactionary approach might be exhibited if the anorexic's own subjective assessment of her disorder was taken into account. It is evident that treatment will be more successful wherever the subject's own context specific understandings of her symptoms are shared with and accepted by the doctor. Sometimes, as Chapter 7 indicates, these understandings may be quite different from the explanatory models held by doctors, researchers and even other anorexics. It is nevertheless essential for successful therapy, that the patient's perspective is taken on board.

The Cognitive Dimensions Supported by the Data in this Book

Control and obsessionalism

I have concentrated so far on summarising findings on clinical dimensions 'disproved' by the data in this book. Other clinical dimensions however were supported by the testimony provided by patients in this study In relation to the dimensions of control and perfectionism/obsessionalism, it seemed that patients did use anorexia as a strategy of obsessive control. It thus appeared that patients' experiences were reflected in these dimensions of clinical knowledge.

Given this finding, it is important to ask why patients exhibited these two clinical symptoms while failing to manifest others. It is not surprising that these dimensions were reported by my sample. Firstly they describe fundamental characteristics reflecting deep-rooted causes and are consequently more subtle and sophisticated constructs than 'fat phobia' or 'fear of maturity'. Secondly, when compared to fat phobia and maturity fear, control and obsessionalism have much more explanatory power. It is theoretically satisfying to suggest that patients develop anorexia because they are dismempowered and wish to regain control. By comparison, the suggestion that sufferers become anorexic 'because they don't want to get fat' is a simplistic evaluation.

Concepts such as control and obsessionalism effectively describe the origins of anorexia. They thus contain a level of generality which make them a vehicle for many more causes than constructs like fat phobia and fear of maturity. However, we should sound a note of caution before uncritically accepting these constructs as entirely accurate reflections of every patient's experience. Patients did describe their anorexia as a strategy of control, but some indicated that they had reached this conclusion as a result of coming to therapy. The book thus concluded that patients may have acquired a clinical vocabulary from clinicians and may use this vocabulary in describing their illness. In the following section, the manner in which the book theorised this process is summarised.

The Sharing of Explanatory Models

Due to improvements in education and mass communication, bio-medical definitions of illness have become disseminated into the general population. The dissemination of medical knowledge has occurred especially in relation to psychiatric disorders such as anorexia. These days, 'folk' explanatory models for such a disorder often contain bio-medical elements. These are frequently derived from magazines, self-help books and counselors (see Chapter 8). In the clinical consultation, for example, the doctor may steer the patient towards a scientific view of her illness.

Scientific theories, however, are also 'part of social reality' (Bourdieu, 1989:18) and may combine with folk theories to produce a socially constructed theory of anorexia. In Chapter 8 patients presented just such an admixture of folk and bio-medical theory in their illness narratives. Significant evidence was presented to demonstrate that narratives were replete with bio-medical references from clinicians, self-help books, and the media. Patients had developed a model of the causes of their disorder based in part on their acquired understanding of the medical model.

Just as patients' understandings of their illness are based largely on bio-medical constructs, so too are clinicians' understandings determined by the society in which they live. As members of the social community, doctors absorb lay understandings of illnesses such as anorexia. 'Seen from this perspective, the professional theory is also a form of lay theory, so that a stringent conceptual dichotomy may be arbitrary' (Lee, 1997:500). In a future study it may be appropriate to evaluate lay and professional views to reveal the common knowledge that surrounds each. This knowledge is an intrinsic element of the social world, and as such is socially determined. As identified in Chapter 1, such knowledge takes different forms during different periods in history (Mannheim, 1952, Elias, 1991). Regardless of its socially constructed and transient nature however, medical knowledge is applied as if it were incontrovertible 'scientific' fact, therefore powerfully eclipsing the less privileged knowledge of the patient.

A more full understanding of the patient's own explanations for the cause of her illness could illuminate the process through which bio-medical theories are assimilated by lay populations. Just as the process by which women have been taught to regard other conditions, (such as menopause), as clinical illnesses, (and have assimilated bio-medical understandings of the menopausal state, Martin, 1987) so too have women absorbed clinical definitions of anorexia. An approach which attends to patients' lay, as well as their clinical, perspective would provide a more holistic understanding of the condition.

Much of the bio-medical knowledge which patients acquire about anorexia is therefore ‘received’. As Chapter 8 of this book suggests, coverage of the disorder in self-help books has increased dramatically in recent years. The remarkable rise in the publicity given to anorexia (Dignon, 2006) may well have helped create the conditions in which the disorder can thrive. Anorexia has therefore been transformed into a ‘popular’ illness. The attention given to the syndrome by academics has also tended to glamourise the disorder. Feminist approaches (Orbach, 1993, MacSween, 1993), for example, often identify the anorexic as a political figure engaged in a struggle for empowerment against the forces of patriarchy. As Swartz (1987) explains, far from being something to avoid ‘having an eating disorder [thus] takes on desirable qualities’ (1987:616). There is a complex fusion of revulsion and fascination that permeates the public perception of anorexia nervosa. This glamourisation of the disorder is often encoded in popular media coverage where celebrities such as Jemima Khan and Calista Flockhart are described as anorexic. While such discourse is couched in cautionary terms, the educative message is expressed in a manner that nonetheless serves to make the condition attractive.

As Swartz explains:

> public education material through television or the print media is [...] almost inevitably followed by an increase in symptoms in patients in treatment [...] if we take the concept of illness negotiation seriously then we must allow that an environment receptive to the understanding of eating disorders may be one in which they will flourish. (1987:617)

It is not surprising then that Murray et al’s (1990) community sample declared that they had gained their understanding of anorexia entirely from the mass media. A similar study by Chiodo and Latimer, (1983), suggests that many bulimics are initiated into the activity through reading a magazine. Some bulimics even suggested that they had acquired eating pathology from consultations with their doctors who questioned them on activities (such as self induced vomiting) they had hitherto not considered.

Other researchers have also expressed concern about the publicising of anorexia. Shorter (1987) for example explains that the increase in specialist anorexia clinics influenced the spread of the illness. Shorter clearly lays the blame for the proliferation of anorexia at the door of the biomedical establishment, who by encoding the disorder as a 'trendy' disease, have clearly contributed to its increase. The medical establishment by promulgating measures ostensibly designed to combat the disorder (such as publicity about its dangers) ironically contributes to its increase. Medicine has therefore effectively created anorexia as a major psychiatric disorder for women (and some men) in the early twenty-first century. Psychiatry has been a key player in maintaining the illness of anorexia in its currently constructed form.

The bio-medical establishment (together with the mass media) have therefore helped to enhance the profile of anorexia as a fashionable disorder. At the same time however, doctors have remained silent concerning their contribution to this process. In particular they exhibit a reluctance to address the socio-cultural prism in which such a proliferation of the disorder has occurred, and their own role in this context. It therefore behoves social researchers to decode the manner in which the psychiatric community, as part of the social world, has plotted the trajectory of the illness. This illness, as constructed by psychiatrists, encompasses both individual distress and social concerns. The beliefs which social actors hold about anorexia and the culturally constituted manner in which they experience and reflect on these beliefs (as observed in the current study) will inevitably influence the causes patients attribute to their symptoms. One of the reasons why anorexia remains rare outside the Western world may be attributed to the absence of 'anorexic' publicity in these countries. Where such publicity is rife, increasing numbers of women articulate their pain through anorexia nervosa. The social construction of anorexia is thus pivotal in determining how and why women experience this disease. The placing of anorexia in its social context is one of the key strengths of the book. An account of further strengths and weaknesses will now be offered.

Strengths and Weaknesses of the Book

Feminism and insights from the field of chronic illness have been applied to the data gathered in this book. The direct application of sociological theory to empirical data represents one of the key strengths of this study. Such an approach links theory with a rigorously gathered set of data, and thus avoids some of the abstraction apparent in earlier studies. A further strength of the study is that it has gathered data from acute patients and has thus provided information about anorexia in its most intense form, enabling more confident conclusions to be drawn from the study's findings. The study also deployed extensive data quality checks, such as triangulation (Denzin, 1989).

While the above represents some of the key strengths of the study there were also areas which would have benefited from further work. Firstly, like all research, the current study was influenced by the 'prejudices' of the researcher. Such 'prejudices' include my left of centre political sympathies and my 'pro-women' approach. These 'personal biases' will have inevitably affected the study's focus and its conclusions should be read in this light. It is impossible to fully suspend such biases, but one can explain them to the reader. The reader is the ultimate judge of the quality of this project, and by being reflexive, I can better enable her (or him) to reach an informed conclusion.

My own prejudices therefore represent one of the limitations of this research. In other, more substantive areas, further limitations may be identified. A closer scrutiny, for example of exactly how patients acquired their understanding of anorexia was needed. It would have been useful, for example, to ask patients directly about their use of anorexic self-help books, magazines and websites. The content of the Day Programme (see page 205) could also have been more closely examined, and its curriculum compared to similar programmes offered elsewhere. In addition, observing the interviews of other doctors would have enabled different physicians' approaches to be compared, allowing me to judge whether these doctors were more (or less) 'directive' than the doctor in the current study. Each of these issues constitutes possible ideas for future work and some further directions in this area will now be offered.

Directions for Future Work

In the concluding chapters of the book, it is important to reflect on the experience of conducting this research. In the process of conducting the study it became evident that several areas for future work had been uncovered. One such area is the study of obesity. While many studies of obesity exist (Fabricatore and Wadden, 2004, Annis et al, 2003, Brownwell and Fairburn, 1995), few investigate 'clinical stereotyping' of the disorder. Like in anorexia, stereotypical constructions of obesity are apparent. Psychiatrists generally suggest that obesity occurs mainly among working class people (Nelson, 1996). This corresponds to the stereotype of the lower class as slothful, indulgent and out of control.[1] As a syndrome, obesity, with its association with instant gratification, corresponds well with prevailing prejudices about working class life. Anorexia, conversely, with its emphasis on self denial and deferred gratification corresponds to stereotypical views of the middle class. In a future project it would be interesting to examine the class profile of a sample of obese people to assess whether such a group really does come predominantly from lower socio-economic strata.

A sociological study of obesity therefore constitutes one area of future research. A further area of future study might centre on the sociology of the body. This book has chosen to focus minimally on the body, instead concentrating on the accuracy and impact of psychiatric 'knowledge' surrounding anorexia. This knowledge has focussed particularly on psychological issues such as obsessionalism,

1 Numerous examples of overweight proletarians can be found in the media, from Harry Enfield's 'Wayne and Waynetta Slob' to the 'Fat slags' comic strip in *Viz*.

control and fear of maturity. The study sought to distance itself from a bodily focus, as it criticises psychiatry for placing a disproportionate emphasis on bodily issues (such as pre-occupation with weight). Anorexia however is quintessentially a bodily (as well as a psychological) disorder. Indeed the knowledge which surrounds anorexia is partly constructed with reference to corporeal issues such as fear of fatness. For this reason, it would be advisable in future studies to analyse data from anorexia patients with reference to sociological work in the area of the body (see Lupton, 1996a, Shilling, 1993).

Conclusion

At the end of this book what have we learned about anorexia nervosa? The key finding of this study is that patients' explanations for their own anorexia must always form the basis of the clinical appraisal, and that the emotions and events which these explanations comprise should be analysed by being set in the social context in which they have occurred. Such an approach has implications for our understanding of the patient, her (or his) illness, and of the society in which that illness occurs. It also has implications for treatment and for approaches to social policy. A women-centred approach to anorexia would involve developing measures which would address women's disempowerment in modern society and the resulting loss of control which women experience (Wingate and Christie, 1978). These measures would incorporate strategies to facilitate equal pay and status, adequate childcare facilities and freedom from sexual and physical abuse.

The practice of bio-medicine is arguably a conservative enterprise. The assessment of anorexia is largely based on communicating the 'right' way of understanding the disorder. Patients acquire a template for assessing their disease (from doctors and the media), and struggle hard to view their illness in the terms laid down in this template. Wanting to get better, they work at understanding anorexia from this perspective. Part of this perspective constructs anorexia as an attempt to avoid fatness. Some patients were angry at biomedicine's view that their illness was simply a diet that had got out of hand. Most patients were very clear that their disorder was a great deal more complicated than this. In disenfranchising patients' explanations, clinicians are stereotyping sufferers. It is interesting to ponder whether such a belittling stereotype would be applied to anorexia if its sufferers were older men instead of young women. These young women sent out a clear message. Anorexia is complicated. If we fail to take this on board, then we are failing anorexic patients. Taking the patient's own perspective into account and placing her at the centre of an appraisal of anorexia, in some measure addresses this complexity. It allows us to better understand the disorder, the patient and the society from which the patient comes.

Appendix: The Eating Disorders Inventory-Adapted (EDI-A)

These questions measure a variety of attitudes, feelings and behaviours. Some of the items relate to food and eating. Others ask you about your feelings about yourself. There are no right or wrong answers so try very hard to be completely honest in your answers. Read each question carefully and tick the answer that best applies to you. Thank you for your co-operation.

	Always	**Usually**	**Often**	**Sometimes**	**Rarely**	**Never**
I feel extremely guilty after over-eating	( )	( )	( )	( )	( )	( )
I am terrified of gaining weight	( )	( )	( )	( )	( )	( )
I am pre-occupied with the desire to be thinner	( )	( )	( )	( )	( )	( )

	Always	Usually	Often	Sometimes	Rarely	Never
If I gain a pound I worry that I will keep gaining	( )	( )	( )	( )	( )	( )
I get confused about what emotions I am feeling	( )	( )	( )	( )	( )	( )
I can clearly identify what emotions I am feeling	( )	( )	( )	( )	( )	( )
I worry that my feelings will get out of control	( )	( )	( )	( )	( )	( )
When I am upset, I don't know if I am sad, frightened or angry	( )	( )	( )	( )	( )	( )

	Always	Usually	Often	Sometimes	Rarely	Never
I have feelings I can't quite identify	( )	( )	( )	( )	( )	( )
When I am upset, I worry that I will start eating	( )	( )	( )	( )	( )	( )
I eat when I am upset	( )	( )	( )	( )	( )	( )
I feel satisfied with the shape of my body	( )	( )	( )	( )	( )	( )
I feel ineffective as a person	( )	( )	( )	( )	( )	( )
I feel alone in the world	( )	( )	( )	( )	( )	( )

	Always	Usually	Often	Sometimes	Rarely	Never
I feel generally in control of things in my life	( )	( )	( )	( )	( )	( )
I wish I were someone else	( )	( )	( )	( )	( )	( )
I have a low opinion about myself	( )	( )	( )	( )	( )	( )
I feel that I am a worth-while person	( )	( )	( )	( )	( )	( )
I feel empty inside (emotionally)	( )	( )	( )	( )	( )	( )
I wish I could return to the security of childhood	( )	( )	( )	( )	( )	( )
I would rather be an adult than a child	( )	( )	( )	( )	( )	( )

	Always	Usually	Often	Sometimes	Rarely	Never
The demands of adulthood are too great	( )	( )	( )	( )	( )	( )
The best years of your life are when you become an adult	( )	( )	( )	( )	( )	( )
Only outstanding performance is good enough in my family	( )	( )	( )	( )	( )	( )
I hate being less than best at things	( )	( )	( )	( )	( )	( )
I am open about my feelings	( )	( )	( )	( )	( )	( )
I trust others	( )	( )	( )	( )	( )	( )
I have close relationships	( )	( )	( )	( )	( )	( )

	Always	Usually	Often	Sometimes	Rarely	Never
I have trouble expressing my emotions to others	( )	( )	( )	( )	( )	( )
I need to keep people at a certain distance (feel uncomfortable if someone tries to get too close)	( )	( )	( )	( )	( )	( )
	( )	( )	( )	( )	( )	( )

That is the end of the questionnaire. Thank you very much for your co-operation.

Bibliography

Acheson, D. (1998), *Independent Inquiry into Inequalities in Health Report*, London: HMSO.

American Psychiatric Association (APA) (1994), *Diagnostic and Statistical Manual of Mental Disorders*, (4th ed.) (DSM-IV), Washington, DC: APA.

—— (1980), *Diagnostic and Statistical Manual of Mental Disorders*, (3rd ed.) (DSM-III), Washington, DC: APA.

—— (1968), *Diagnostic and Statistical Manual of Mental Disorders*, (2nd ed.) (DSM-II), Washington, DC: APA.

Anderson, R., Bury, M. (1988), *Living with Chronic Illness*, Unwin Hyman: London.

Annandale, E. (1998), *The Sociology of Health and Medicine: A Critical Introduction*, Cambridge: Polity.

Annis, M., Cash, N., Thomas, F., Hrabosky, I. J. (2003). *Body Image and Psychosocial Differences Among Stable Average Weight, Currently Overweight, and Formerly Overweight Women: the Role of Stigmatizing Experiences*. New York: Elsevier Ltd.

Armstrong, D. (1995), The rise of surveillance medicine, *The Sociology of Health and Illness*, 17, 3, 393–404.

—— (1982), The Doctor-Patient Relationship: 1930–1980. In Wright, P., Treacher, A. (eds.) *The Problem of Medical Knowledge: Examining the Social Construction of Medicine* (49–68) Southampton: Edinburgh University Press.

Atkinson, P. (1983), Eating Virtue. In Murcott, A. (ed.) *The Sociology of Food and Eating* (9–17) Aldershot: Gower.

Azuma, Y., Henmi, M. (1982), A Study on the Incidence of Anorexia Nervosa in School Girls, *Annual Report of the Research Group in Eating Disorders, Japan*, 30–4.

Banks, C. G. (1992), Culture in Culture-Bound Syndromes: The Case of Anorexia Nervosa, *Social Science and Medicine*, 34, 8, 867–84.

Bayer, R. (1987), *Homosexuality and American Psychiatry: The Politics of Diagnosis*, New York: Basic Books.

Beck, U. (1992), *Risk Society*, London: Sage, cited in Annandale, E. (1998), *The Sociology of Health and Medicine: A Critical Introduction*, Cambridge: Polity.

Beech, H. R. (1978), *Behavioural Treatment of Obsessional States*, Chichester: Wiley.

Belenky, M. F., McVicker-Clinchy, B., Goldberger, N. R., Tarule, J. M. (1986), *Women's Ways of Knowing: the Development of Self, Voice and Mind*, New York: Basic Books.

Berg, M., Mol, A. (1998), *Differences in Medicine: Unravelling Practices, Techniques and Bodies*, London: Duke University Press.

Berger P., Luckmann, T. (1966), *The Social Construction of Reality*, New York: Penguin.

Bernstein, B. (1971), *Class, Codes and Control*, London: Routledge and Kegan Paul.

Biddle, B. J. (2001), *Social Class, Poverty and Education*, London: Routledge.

Blaxter, M. (1981), *The Health of the Children: A Review of Research on the Place of Health in Cycles of Disadvantage*, London: Heinemann.

——, Patterson, E. (1983), The Goodness is Out of It: The Meaning of Food to Two Generations. In Murcott, A. (ed.) *The Sociology of Food and Eating* (95–105) Aldershot: Gower.

Bordo, S. (1993), *Unbearable Weight: Feminism, Western Culture and the Body*, Berkeley: University of California Press.

—— (1988), Anorexia Nervosa: Psychopathology as the Crystallization of Culture. In Diamond, I., Quinby, L. (eds.) *Feminism and Foucault:Reflections on Resistance* (87–117), West Hannover, Mass: Northeastern University Press.

Boskind-White, M., White, W. C. (1986), Bulimarexia: A Historical-Sociocultural Perspective. In Brownwell, K., Foreyt, J. (eds.) *Handbook of Eating Disorder* (353–66), New York: Basic Books.

Bourdieu, P. (1996), *The State Nobility*, Oxford: Blackwell.

—— (1994), *Distinction*, (2nd ed.) Cambridge, Mass: Harvard University Press.

—— (1989), Social Space and Symbolic Power, *Sociological Theory*, 7, 14–25.

—— (1984), *Distinction*, (1st ed.) London: Routledge.

Bourgeault, I. L., Armstrong, P., Armstrong, H., Choiniere, J., Lexchin, J., Mykhalovskiy, E., Peters, S., White, J. (2001), Everyday Experiences of Implicit Rationing: Comparing the Voices of Nurses in California and British Columbia, *Sociology of Health and Illness*, 23, 5, 633–53.

Bowling, A. (1997), *Research Methods in Health*, Milton Keynes: Open University.

Broverman, I. K., Vogel, S.R., Broverman, D., Clarkson, F. E., Rosenkrantz, P. S. (1972), Sex Role Stereotypes: A Current Appraisal, *Journal of Social Issues*, 28, 59–78.

Brownwell, D. K., Fairburn, G. C. (1995), *Eating Disorders and Obesity: A Comprehensive Handbook*, New York: The Guilford Press.

Bruch, H. (1979), *The Golden Cage: the Enigma of Anorexia*, New York: Vintage Books.

—— (1978), *The Golden Cage: the Enigma of Anorexia*, Wells: Open Books.

—— (1973), *Eating Disorders*, New York: Basic Books.

Brumberg, J. J. (1988a), *Fasting Girls: the History of Anorexia Nervosa*, New York: Vintage books.

—— (1988b), *Fasting Girls: The Emergence of Anorexia Nervosa as a Modern Disease*, Cambridge, MA.: Havard University Press.

Buckroyd, J. (1996), *Anorexia and Bulimia: Your Questions Answered*, Shaftsbury: Element.

Burgoyne, J., Clarke, D. (1983), You Are What You Eat: Food and Family Reconstruction. In Murcott, A. (ed.) *The Sociology of Food and Eating* (152–63) Aldershot: Gower.

Burke, P. (2000), *A Social History of Knowledge: from Gutenberg to Diderot*, Cambridge: Polity.

Burns, N., Grove, S.K. (1993), *The Practice of Nursing Research: Conduct, Critique and Utilization*, (2nd ed.) Philadelphia: Saunders.

Bury, M. (2001), Illness narratives: fact or fiction?, *Sociology of Health & Illness*, 23, 3, 263–85.

—— (1991), The sociology of chronic illness: A review of research and prospects, *Sociology of Health and Illness*, 13,4, 451–68.

—— (1988), Meanings at Risk: the experience of arthritis. In Anderson, R., Bury, M., (eds.), (1988), *Living with Chronic Illness*, (89–116), Unwin Hyman: London.

—— (1982), Chronic Illness as Biographical Disruption, *Sociology of Health and Illness*, 4, 167–82.

Bush, H., Williams, R., Bradby, H., Anderson, A., Lean, M. (1998), Family Hospitality and Ethnic Tradition among South Asian, Italian and General Population Women in the West of Scotland, *The Sociology of Health and Illness*, 20 (3): 351–80.

Callaghan, S., Joseph, S. (1995), Self Concept and Peer Victimization among School Children, *Personality and Individual Differences*, 18 (1), 161–3.

Callender, C. (1996), Women and Employment. In Hallet C. (ed.) *Women and Social Policy* (31–51), London: Prentice Hall.

Cantrell, P. J., Ellis, J. B. (1991), Gender Role and Risk Patterns for Eating Disorders in Men and Women, *Journal of Clinical Psychology*, 47, 1, 53–7.

Caplan, P. J. (1990), Making Mother Blaming Visible: The Emperor's New Clothes, *Women and Therapy*, 10, 1–2, 61–70.

Carlos, A. L. (1972), Psychiatry in Latin America, *British Journal of Psychiatry*, 121, 121–36.

Chalker, R. (2000), *The Clitoral Truth: the World at Your Fingertips*, New York: Seven Stories Press.

Charles, N., Kerr, M. (1988), *Women, Food and Families*, Manchester: Manchester University Press.

Chernin, K. (1986), *Women, Eating and Identity*, London: Virago.

Chiodo, J., Latimer, P. R. (1983), Vomiting as a Learned Weight Control Technique in Bulimia, *Journal of Behaviour Therapy and Experimental Psychiatry*, 14, 131–5.

Chitty, C. (2002), Education and Social Class, *The Political Quarterly*, 73, 2, 208–10.

Collins, H., Pinch, T. (1994) *The Golem: What You Should Know About Science*, Cambridge: Cambridge University Press.

Comaroff, J. (1982), Medicine: Symbol and Ideology. In Wright, P., Treacher, A. (eds.) *The Problem of Medical Knowledge: Examining the Social Construction of Medicine* (49–68) Southampton: Edinburgh University Press.

Costin, C. (1997), *The Eating Disorders Sourcebook*, Los Angeles: Lowell House.

Council of Heads of Medical Schools Website, (2005): http://www.chms.ac.uk

Crisp, A. H. (1995), *Anorexia Nervosa: Let Me Be*, Hove: Lawrence Erlbaum.

——, Palmer, R. L., Kalucy, R. S. (1976), How Common is Anorexia Nervosa? A Prevalence Study, *British Journal of Psychiatry*, 128, 549–54.

Crompton, R. (1998), *Class and Stratification: An Introduction to current debates* (2nd ed.), Cambridge: Polity.

Crozier, W. R., Skliopidou, E. (2002), Adult Recollections of Name Calling at School, *Educational Psychology*, 22 (1), 113–24.

Davis, E. C. (1995), Early and On-time Puberty and the Relationship to Anorexia, Bulimia and Obesity, *Dissertation of Abstracts International, Section A-Humanities and Social Sciences*, May, 55, 3414.

Denzin, N. (1989), *The Research Act*, New Jersey: Prentice Hall.

—— (1970), *Sociological Methods: A Sourcebook*, London: Butterworths.

Department for Education and Employment (DofE) (2000), *Education and Training Statistics for the United Kingdom*, London: HMSO.

—— (1996), *Education Statistics for the United Kingdom, 1995*, London: HMSO.

DeVault, M. (1991), *Feeding the Family: the social organisation of caring as gendered work*, Chicago: University Press.

Dey, I. (1993) *Qualitative Data Analysis: A User-friendly guide for Social Scientists* London: Routledge.

Dignon, A. (2006), The Anorexic stereotype: A Sociological Critique of the Medical Construction of Anorexia, PhD Thesis, University of Leicester.

——, Beardsmore, A., Spain, S., Kuan, A. (2006), Why I won't eat: patient testimony from 15 anorexics concerning the causes of their disorder, *Journal of Health Psychology*, 11,6,942–56.

Dolan, B., Lacey, J. H., Evans, C. (1990), Eating Behaviour and Attitudes to Weight and Shape in British Women from Three Ethnic Groups, *British Journal of Psychiatry*, 157, 523–8.

Douglas, M. (1972), Deciphering a Meal, *Daedalus*,101 (1), 61–81.

Eagles, J. H.,Wilson, A. M., Hunter, D., Callender, J. S. (1990), A comparison of anorexia nervosa and affective psychosis in young females, *Psychological Medicine*, 20, 119–23.

Ehrenreich, B., English, D. (1989) *For Her Own Good: 150 Years of the Expert's Advice to Women*, New York: Anchor Books.

Elias, N. (1991), *The Symbol Theory*, London: Sage.

—— (1978), *The Civilizing Process*, Oxford: Blackwell.

Ellis, R. (1983), The Way to a Man's Heart: Food in the Violent Home. In Murcott, A. (ed.) *The Sociology of Food and Eating* (164–71) Aldershot: Gower.

Elston, M. (1997) (ed), *The Sociology of Medical Science and Technology*, Oxford: Blackwell.

Fabrega, H. F. (1974), *Disease and Social Behaviour*, Cambridge, Mass: Massachusetts Institute of Technology Press.

Fabricatore, N. A., Wadden, A. T. (2004), *Psychological Aspects of Obesity*, New York: Elsevier Ltd.

Fallon, P., Katzman, M., Wooley, S. C. (1994), (eds.) *Feminist Perspectives in Eating Disorders*, New York: Guildford.

Fatout, M. F. (1993), Physically Abused Children: Activity as a Therapeutic Medium, *Social Work with Groups*, 1993, 16 (3), 83–96.

Finkelhor, D. (1981), *Sexually Victimized Children*, London: The Free Press, MacMillan.

Fischler, C. (1980), Food habits, social change and the nature/culture dilemma, *Social Science Information*, 19, 6, 937–53.

Fisher, S. (2001), *In the Patient's Best Interest*, Rutgers: New Brunswick.

Foster, J. (2001), *Data Analysis Using SPSS for Windows, versions 8 to 10: A beginner's guide*, London: Sage.

Foucault, M. (1986), Nietzche, Genealogy, History. In Rabinow, P. (ed.) *The Foucault Reader* (76–100) Harmondsworth: Penguin.

—— (1979), *Discipline and Punish, the Birth of the Prison*, London: Penguin.

Fox-Keller, E. (1985) *Reflections on Gender and Science*, New York: Yale University Press.

Frasciello, L. M., Willard, S. G. (1995), Anorexia Nervosa in Males: A Case Report and Review of the Literature, *Clinical Social Work Journal*, 23 (1), 47–58.

Freidson, E. (1970a), *The Profession of Medicine*, New York: Dodd, Mead and Co.

—— (1970b), *Professional Dominance: The Social Structure of Medical Care*, New York: Atherton.

Gahan, C., Hannibal, M. (1998), *Doing Qualitative Research using QSR NUD*IST*, London: Sage.

Gard, M. C., Freeman, C. P. (1996), The Dismantling of a Myth: A Review of Eating Disorders and Socio-economic Status, *International Journal of Eating Disorders*, 20, 1–12.

Garfinkel, P. (1992), Classification and Diagnosis. In Halmi, K. A. (ed.) *Psychobiology and Treatment of Anorexia Nervosa and Bulima Nervosa* (37–60) Washington: American Psychiatric Press.

Garner, D. M., Garfinkel, P. E. (1980), Socio-Cultural Factors in the Development of Anorexia, *Psychological Medicine*, 10, 647–56.

—— (1979), The Eating Attitudes Test: An Index of the Symptoms of Anorexia Nervosa, *Psychological Medicine*, 9, 273–9.

——, Schwartz, D., Thompson, M. (1980), Cultural Expectations of thinness in Women, *Psychological Reports*, 47, 483–91.

——, Olmstead, M. P. (1983a), An Overview of Socio-Cultural factors in the development of Anorexia Nervosa. In Darby, P. L. (ed.) *Anorexia Nervosa: Recent developments in Research* (65–82) New York: Alan R. Liss.

Garner, D. M., Olmstead, M. P., Polivy, J. (1983b), Development and Validation of a Multi-dimensional Eating Disorder Inventory for Anorexia Nervosa and Bulimia, *International Journal of Eating Disorders*, 2, 15–34.

Gelder, M. G., Gath, D., Mayou, R. (1983) *Oxford Textbook of Psychiatry*, Oxford: Oxford University Press.

Gelder, M. G., Lopez-Ibor, J. L., Andreasen, N., (2000) *New Oxford Textbook of Psychiatry*, Oxford: Oxford University Press.

Gelder, M. G., Mayou, R., Cohen, P. (2004), *Shorter Oxford Textbook of Psychiatry*, Oxford: Oxford University Press.

German, G. A. (1972), Aspects of Clinical Psychiatry in Sub-Saharan Africa, *British Journal of Psychiatry*, 121, 461–79.

Germov, J., Williams, L. (2004), *A Sociology of Food and Nutrition: The Social Appetite*, (2nd ed.), Melbourne: Oxford University Press.

Giddens, A. (1991), *Modernity and Self Identity*, Cambridge: Polity.

Goffman, E. (1968), *Asylums: Essays on the Social Situation of Mental Patients and Other Inmates*, Harmondsworth: Penguin.

—— (1963), *Stigma: Notes on the Management of a Spoiled Identity*, New York: Prentice Hall.

Gower, S., McMahon J. B. (1989), Social Class and Prognosis in Anorexia Nervosa, *International Journal of Eating Disorders*, 8, 1, 105–9.

Graham, H. (1984), *Women, Health and the Family*, Brighton: Harvester Wheatsheaf.

Gregurek, R. (1994), Anorexia Nervosa in Males: the Question of Disturbed Gender Identity, *Psychiatrica Danubina*, 6, 1–2, 109–11.

Griffiths, L. (2001), Categorizing to Exclude: the Discursive Construction of Cases in Community Mental Health Teams, *Sociology of Health and Illness*, 23, 5, 678–700.

Grolnick, W. S., Gurland, S. T. (2002), Mothering: Retrospect and Prospect. In McHale, J. P., Grolnick, W. S. (eds.) *Retrospect and Prospect in the Psychological Study of Families* (5–33), Mahwah, New Jersey: Lawrence Erlbaum.

Habermas, T., (1991), The role of psychiatric and medical traditions in the discovery of anorexia nervosa in France, Germany and Italy 1873–1918, *Journal of Nervous Mental Diseases*, 179, 4, 360–4.

Habermas, J. (1970) *Toward a Rational Society*, Boston, MA: Beacon Press.

Hallet, C. (1996), *Women and Social Policy*, London: Prentice Hall.

Halmi, K. A., Casper, R. C., Eckhert, E. D., Goldberg, S. C., Davis, J. M. (1979), Unique Features Associated with Age of Onset of Anorexia Nervosa, *Psychiatry Research*, 1, 209–15.

Hamburg, P., Herzog, D. B. (1985), Studying Reports of Women Medical Students on their Eating Disorders, *Journal of Medical Education*, 60, 644–6.

Harding, S. (1991) *Whose Science Whose Knowledge*?, Milton Keynes: Open University Press.

Health Education Council (1983), *A Discussion Paper on Proposals for Nutritional Guidelines for Health Education in Britain (NACNE)*, London: Health Education Council.

Heebink, D. M., Sunday, S. R., Halmi, K. A. (1995), Anorexia Nervosa and Bulimia Nervosa in Adolescence: Effects of Age and Menstrual Status on Psychological Variables, *Journal of Academic Child and Adolescent Psychiatry*, 34, 3, 378–82.

Helman, C. G. (2000), *Culture, Health and Illness*, (4th ed.) Oxford: Butterworth-Heinemann.

—— (1987), Heart Disease and the Cultural Construction of Time: The Type A Behaviour Pattern as a Western Culture Bound Syndrome, *Social Science and Medicine*, 25, 9, 969–79.

Hepworth, J. (2004), The Social Construction of Eating Disorders. In Germov, J., Williams, L. (eds.), *A Sociology of Food and Nutrition: The Social Appetite*, (2nd ed.) (368–82), Oxford University Press: Melbourne.

—— (1999), *The Social Construction of Anorexia Nervosa*, London: Sage.

Herzog, D. B., Norman, D. K., Gordon, C., Pepose, M. (1984), Sexual Conflict and Eating Disorders in Twenty-seven Males, American Journal of Psychiatry, 141, 989–90.

Hewitt-Taylor, J. (2001), Use of Constant Comparative Analysis in Qualitative Research, *Nursing Standard* 15:42, 39–42.

Higgs, P. (2003), The Limits and Boundaries of Medical Knowledge. In Scambler, G. (ed.) Sociology as Applied to Medicine, (181–91) Saunders: Edinburgh.

Hindler, C. G., Crisp, A. H., McGuigan, S., Joughin, J. (1994), Anorexia Nervosa: Change over Time in Age of Onset, Presentation and Duration of Illness, *Psychological Medicine*, 24, 719–29.

Hinton, P. R. (2000), *Stereotypes, Cognition and Culture*, Hove: Psychology Press.

Hoek, H. W. (1993), Review of the Epidemiological Studies of Eating Disorders, *International Review of Psychiatry*, 5, 61–74.

—— (1991), The Incidence and Prevalence of Anorexia Nervosa and Bulimia Nervosa in Primary Care, *Psychological Medicine*, 21, 455–60.

——, Brook, F. G. (1985), Patterns of Care in Anorexia Nervosa, *Journal of Psychiatric Research*, 19, 155–60.

Holton, R. J., Turner, B. S. (1986), *Talcott Parsons on Economy and Society*, London: Routledge.

Hsu, L. K. G., Crisp, A. H., Callender, J. S. (1992), Recovery in Anorexia Nervosa: The Patient's Perspective, *International Journal of Eating Disorders*, 11, 341–50.

Ilmonen, K. (1991), Change and stability in Finnish eating habits. In Furst, E., Prattalla, R., Eckstrom, M., Holm, L., Kjaernes, K. (eds.), *Palatable worlds: socio cultural food studies*, (169–84), Solum Forlag: Oslo.

Irigaray, L. (1985), *This Sex Which is Not One*, Ithaca: Cornell University Press.

Jewson, N. (1976), The disappearance of the sick man from medical cosmology, *Sociology*, 10:225–44.

Jones, K. (1991), *The Making of Social Policy in Britain*, London: Athlone.

Jobling, R. (1988), The experience of psoriasis under treatment. In Anderson, R., Bury, M. (eds.), (1988), *Living with Chronic Illness*, (225–44), Unwin Hyman: London.

Kaplan, H., Sadock, B. (1995), *Comprehensive Textbook of Psychiatry, VI*, (6th ed.) Baltimore: Willams and Wilkins.

—— (1985), *Comprehensive Textbook of Psychiatry, IV*, (4th ed.) Baltimore: Willams and Wilkins.

—— (1967), *Comprehensive Textbook of Psychiatry, I*, (1st ed.) Baltimore: Willams and Wilkins.

Katzman, M. A. (1993), Women in Groups. Experiments in Taking up Space. Plenary address presented at the National Association of Anorexia Nervosa and Associated Disorders. *National Eating Disorders Conference*, Chicago, Illinois, April 19–21, 1993.

——, Lee, S. (1997), Beyond Body Image: The Integration of Feminist and Transcultural Theories in the Understanding of Self Starvation, *International Journal of Eating Disorders*, 22, 385–94.

Kelly, M. P., Field, D. (1996), Medical Sociology, Chronic Illness and the Body, *Sociology of Health and Illness*, 18, 2, 241–57.

Kleinman, A., (1988), *The Illness Narratives: Suffering, Healing and the Human Condition*, Basic Books, New York.

Kristeva, J. (2001), Experiencing the Phallus as Extraneous: Women's Twofold Oedipus Complex. In Hartocollis, P. (ed.) *Mankind's Oedipal Destiny: Libidinal and Aggressive Aspects of Sexuality* (37–53) Madison: International Universities Press.

Kuhn (1996), *The Structure of Scientific Revolutions*, Chicago: University of Chicago Press.

Kutchins, H., Kirk, S. A. (1997), *Making Us Crazy: DSM- The Psychiatric Bible and the Creation of Mental Disorders*, London: Constable.

Lawrence, M. (1998), *The Anorexic Experience*, (3rd ed) London: Women's Press.

—— (1995), *The Anorexic Experience*, (2nd ed.) London: Women's Press.

—— (1984), *The Anorexic Experience*, (1st ed.) London: Women's Press.

Lee, S. (1997), How Lay is Lay? Chinese Students Perceptions of Anorexia Nervosa in Hong Kong, *Social Science and Medicine*, 44, 4, 491–502.

—— (1996), Reconsidering the Status of Anorexia Nervosa as a Culture-Bound Syndrome, *Social Science and Medicine*, 42, 21–34.

—— (1995), Self-starvation in Context: Towards a Culturally Sensitive Understanding of Anorexia Nervosa, *Social Science and Medicine*, 41, 1, 25–36.

—— (1991), Anorexia Nervosa in Hong Kong: a Chinese Perspective, *Psychological Medicine*, 1991, 21, 703–11.

Levenkron, S. (2000), *Anatomy of Anorexia*, London: Norton.

Leyens, J. P., Yzerbyt, V., Schadron, G. (1994), *Stereotypes and Social Cognition*, London: Sage.

Light, D., Hughes, D. (2001), Introduction: A Sociological Perspective on Rationing: Power, Rhetoric and Situated Practices, *Sociology of Health and Illness*, 23, 5, 551–69.

Lindsay, C. (2000), *Conquering Anorexia*, Chichester: Summerdale.

Locker, D. (2003), Living with Chronic Illness. In Scambler, G. (ed.) *Sociology as Applied to Medicine*, (78–91) Saunders: Edinburgh.

—— (1983) *Disability and Disadvantage: The Consequences of Chronic Illness*, Tavistock, London.

Lofland, J., Lofland, L. (1995), *Analysing Social Settings: a guide to qualitative observation and analysis*, (3rd ed.) Belmont, CA: Wadsworth.

Lucas, A. R., Beard, C. M., O'Fallon, W. M., Kurland, L. T. (1988), Anorexia Nervosa in Rochester, Minnesota: a 45 year study, *Mayo Clinic Proceedings*, 63, 433–42.

Lupton D. (1996a), *Food, The Body and the Self*, London: Sage.

—— (1996b), *Medicine as Culture* (2nd ed.), London: Sage.

—— (1994), *Medicine as Culture*, London: Sage.

MacDonald, L. (1988), The experience of stigma: Living with rectal cancer. In Anderson, R., Bury, M. (eds), (1988), *Living with Chronic Illness*, (177–202), Unwin Hyman: London.

MacCrae, C.N., Stangor, C., Hewstone, M. (1996), *Stereotypes and Stereotyping*, New York: Guildford Press.

Mackler, B. (1976), The Mother Blamers, *Clinical Psychologist*, 30,1, 9–11.

MacSween, M. (1993), *Anorexic Bodies: a Feminist and Sociological Account of Anorexia Nervosa*, London: Routledge.

Malos, E. (1980), *The Politics of Housework*, London: Allison and Busby.

Malson, H. (1992), Anorexia Nervosa: Displacing Universalities and Replacing Gender. In Nicholson, P., Ussher, J. (eds.) *The Psychology of Women's Health and Health Care* (62–91) London: Macmillan.

Mannheim, K. (1952), *Essay on the Sociology of Knowledge*, London: Routledge and Kegan Paul.

Marsh, C. (1994), Sexual Assault and Domestic Violence in the African American Community, *Western Journal of Black Studies*, 17, 3, 149–55.

Martin, E. (1987), *The Woman in the Body*, Milton Keynes: Open University Press.

Mason, J. (2003) *Qualitative Researching*, (2nd ed.), London: Sage.

McCallum, I., Demie, F. (2001), Social Class, Ethnicity and Educational Performance, *Educational Research*, 43, 2, 147–60.

Mennell, S. (2004) Foreword. In Germov, J., Williams, L. (2004), *A Sociology of Food and Nutrition: The Social Appetite*, (2nd ed.) Oxford University Press: Melbourne.

—— (1996) *All Manners of Food*, University of Illinois Press: Chicago.

——, Murcott, A., Van Otterloo, A. H. (1994), *The Sociology of Food, Eating, Diet and Culture*, London: Sage.

Miller, G. W. (1970), Factors in School Achievement and Social Class, *Journal of Educational Psychology*, 61, 4, 260–9.

Minuchin, S. (1991), *Families and Family Therapy*, London: Routledge.

——, Rosman, B. L., Baker, L. (1978), *Psychosomatic Families: Anorexia Nervosa in Context*, Cambridge, Mass: Havard University Press.

Mishler, E. (1984), *The Discourse of Medicine: Dialectics of Medical Interviews*, New Jersey: Ablex.

Mizrachi, N. (2002), Epistemology and Legitimacy in the Production of Anorexia Nervosa in the Journal Psychosomatic Medicine 1939–1979, *Sociology of Health and Illness*, 24, 4, 462–90.

Morgan H. G., Russell, G. F. M. (1975), Value of Family Background and Clinical Features as Predictors of Long-term Outcome in Anorexia Nervosa: Four Year Follow-up Study of 41 Patients, *Psychological Medicine*, 5, 355–71.

Murcott, A. (1983), (ed.) *The Sociology of Food and Eating*, Aldershot: Gower.

Murray, S., Touyz, S., Beaumont, P. (1990), Knowledge about Eating Disorders in the Community, *International Journal of Eating Disorders*, 9, 87–93.

Nadoka, T., Oiji, A., Takahashi, S., Morioka,Y., Kashiwakura, M., Totsuka, S. (1996), An Epidemiological Study of Eating Disorders in a Northern Area of Japan, *Acta Psychiatrica Scandinavica*, 93, 305–10.

Neki, J. S. (1973), Psychiatry in South East Asia, *British Journal of Psychiatry*, 123, 257–69.

Nelson, S.L. (1996), Relative Body Weight among Black American Women: Relationships to Acculturation, Social Class, Attitudes and Perceived Power, *Dissertation of Abstracts International; Section B: The Sciences and Engineering*, 57(6-B), 4036.

Nettleton, S. (1995), *The Sociology of Health and Illness*, Cambridge: Polity.

Oakley, A. (1992), *Social Support and Motherhood*, Oxford: Blackwell.

—— (1987), From Walking Wombs to Test-tube Babies. In Stanworth, M. (ed.) *Reproductive Technologies: Gender, Motherhood and Medicine* (36–56) Cambridge: Polity.

—— (1976) *Housewife*, Harmondsworth: Penguin.

Olweus, D. (1995), Bullying or Peer Abuse at School: Facts and Interventions, *Current Directions in Psychological Science*, 4, 6, 196–200.

O'Neil, M. L., Kerig, P. K. (2000), Attributions of Self Blame and Perceived Control as Moderators of Adjustment in Battered Women, *Journal of Interpersonal Violence*, 15, 10, 1036–49.

OPCS (1997), *1991 Census: Key Statistics for Urban and Rural Areas*, London: HMSO.
—— (1993), *1991 Census Report for Great Britain*, London: HMSO.
—— (1980), *Classification of Occupations 1980*, London: HMSO.
Orbach, S. (1993), *Hunger Strike: the Anorectic's Struggle as a Metaphor for Our Age*, (2nd ed.) London: Penguin.
Palmer, R. L. (1989), *Anorexia Nervosa: A Guide for Sufferers and their Families*, Harmondsworth: Penguin.
——, Oppenheimer, R., Chaloner, D. A., Dignon, A. M., Howells, K. (1990), Childhood Sexual Experiences with Adults reported by Women with Eating Disorders, *British Journal Of Psychiatry*, 699–703.
Parry-Jones, W. (1985), Archival exploration of anorexia nervosa, *Journal of Psychiatric Research*, 1985, 9, (2–3), 95–100.
Parsons, T. (1951), Illness and the Role of the Physician: a Sociological Perspective. In Stoeckle, J. D. (1987) (ed.) *Encounters between Patients and Doctors:An Anthology* (147–56) Cambridge Massachusetts: MIT Press.
Pickering, M. (2001), *Stereotyping: the politics of representation*, Basingstoke: Palgrave.
Platt, S., Thomas, H. (1993), Introduction. In Platt, S., Thomas, H., Scott, S.,Williams, G. (1993) (eds.) *Locating Health: Sociological and Historical Explorations*, Aldershot: Avebury.
——, Scott, S., Williams, G. (1993) (eds.) *Locating Health: Sociological and Historical Explorations*, Aldershot: Avebury.
Polit D., Hungler B. (1997), *Essentials of Nursing Research: Methods, Appraisal and Utilization*, Philadelphia: Lippincott.
—— (1995), *Nursing Research: Principles and Methods*, Philadelphia: Lippincott.
Pope, C., Mays, N., (2000) *Qualitative Research in Healthcare*, London: BMJ publications.
Porter, R. (2002), *Madness: A Brief History*, Oxford: Oxford University Press.
Prince, R. (1985), The Concept of Culture Bound Syndromes: Anorexia Nervosa and Brain Fag, *Social Science and Medicine*, 21, 2, 197–203.
Radley, A. (1994), *Making Sense of Illness: The Social Psychology of Health and Disease*, Sage: London.
Rastam, M., Gillberg, C. (1991), The Family Background in Anorexia Nervosa: A Population Based Study, *Journal of American Academic and Child Adolescent Psychiatry*, 30, 2, 283–9.
——, Garton, M. (1989), Anorexia Nervosa in a Swedish Urban Region: a Population Based Study, *British Journal Of Psychiatry*, 155, 642–6.
Rathner, G., Messner, K. (1993), Detection of Eating Disorders in a Small Rural Town: an Epidemiological Study, *Psychological Medicine*, 23, 175–84.

Raymond, N. C., Mitchell , J. E., Fallon, P., Katzman, M. A. (1994), A Collaborative Approach to the use of Medication. In Fallon, P., Katzman, M., Wooley, S. C. (eds.) *Feminist Perspectives in Eating Disorders* (231–50) New York: Guildford.

Rhodes, G. (2001) *The Complete Rhodes around Britain*, BBC Consumer Publishing: London.

Ritzenbaugh, C. (1982), Obesity as a Culture Bound Syndrome, *Culture, Medicine and Psychiatry*, 6, 347–61.

Ritzer, G. (1996), *The MacDonaldization of Society*, Pine Forge Press: Thousand Oaks, California.

Robinson, P. H., Holden, N. L. (1986), Bulima Nervosa in the Male: a Report of Nine Cases, *Psychological Medicine*, 16, 795–803.

Rogers, L., Resnick, M. D., Mitchell, J. E., Blum, R. W. (1997), The Relationship between Socio-economic status and Eating Disordered Behaviours in a Community Sample of Adolescent Girls, *International Journal of Eating Disorders*, 22, 15–23.

Rowe, D. (1997) Introduction. In Kutchins, H., Kirk, S. A. (1997), *Making Us Crazy: DSM-The Psychiatric Bible and the Creation of Mental Disorders,* London: Constable.

Royal College of Physicians (2004), *Storing Up Problems, The medical case for a slimmer nation: Report of a working party of the Royal College of Physicians, Royal College of Pediatric and Child Health and the faculty of Public Health Medicine*, Royal College of Physicians: London.

Ruskay-Rabinor, J. (1994) Mothers, Daughters and Eating Disorders: Honoring the Mother-Daughter Relationship. In Fallon, P., Katzman, M., Wooley, S. C. (eds.) *Feminist Perspectives in Eating Disorders* (272–86) New York: Guildford.

Russell, G. F. M., (2000), Disorders of Eating, In Gelder, M. G., Lopez-Ibor, J. L., Andreasen, N. (2000) *New Oxford Textbook of Psychiatry*, (835–43), Oxford: Oxford University Press.

—— (1970), Anorexia Nervosa: its Identity as an Illness and its Treatment. In Price, J. K. (ed.) Modern Trends in Psychological Medicine, London: Butterworth, cited in Halmi, K. A. (1992) *Psychobiology and Treatment of Anorexia Nervosa and Bulima Nervosa,* Washington: American Psychiatric Press.

Ryle, J. A. (1936) Anorexia Nervosa, *Lancet*, ii, 893–9.

Sackett, D. L., Scott Richardson, W., Rosenberg, W. M. Haynes, R. B. (1997) *Evidence based medicine: How to practice and teach EBM*, London: Churchill Livingstone.

Sands, R., Tricker, J., Sherman, C., Armatas, C., Maschette, W. (1997), Disordered Eating Patterns, Body Image, Self-esteem and Physical Activity in Pre-adolescent School Children, *International Journal of Eating Disorders*, 21, 2, 159–66.

Scambler, G. (2003a) *Sociology as Applied to Medicine*, Saunders: Edinburgh.

—— (2003b) Deviance, Sick Role and Stigma. In Scambler, G. (ed.) *Sociology as Applied to Medicine*, (192–202), Saunders: Edinburgh.

——, Hopkins, A. (1988) Accommodating epilepsy in families. In Anderson, R., Bury, M. (eds), (1988), *Living with Chronic Illness*, (156–76), Unwin Hyman: London.

Scull, A. T. (1982), *Museums of Madness*, London: Penguin.

Seale, C. (2000) *The Quality of Qualitative Research*, London: Sage.

——, Pattison, S., Davey, B. (2001) *Medical Knowledge: Doubt and Certainty*, Buckingham: Open University Press.

Sesan, R. (1994), Feminist Inpatient Treatment for Eating Disorders: An Oxymoron. In Fallon, P., Katzman, M., Wooley, S. C. (eds.) *Feminist Perspectives in Eating Disorders* (251–71) New York: Guildford.

Sheehan, H. L., Summers, V. K. (1949) The syndrome of hypopituitarism, *American Journal of Medicine*, 18, 319–78

Sheldon, J. H. (1939), Anorexia Nervosa, *Proceedings of the Royal Society of Medicine*, 32, 738–41.

Shorter, E. (1987), The First Great Increase in Anorexia Nervosa, *Journal of Social History*, 21, 69–79.

Showalter, E. (1987), *The Female Malady: Women, Madness and English Culture 1830–1980*, London: Virago.

Sigerist, H. E. (1933), *The Great Doctors*, New York: Norton.

Silverman, D. (2004) *Qualitative Research, Theory, Method and Practice*, London: Sage.

—— (2000) *Doing Qualitative Research*, London: Sage.

—— (1987), Communication and Medical Practice: Social Relations in the Clinic, London: Sage, cited in Lupton, D. (1994) *Medicine as Culture*, London: Sage.

Simoni, J. M., Ng, M. T. (2002), Abuse, Health Locus of Control and Perceived Health among HIV Positive Women, *Health Psychology*, 21, 1, 89–93.

Slater, E., Roth, M. (1969), Clinical Psychiatry, London: Tindall and Cassell, cited in Kutchins, H., Kirk, S. A. (1997), *Making Us Crazy: DSM- The Psychiatric Bible and the Creation of Mental Disorders*, London: Constable.

Stacey, M. (1988), *The Sociology of Health and Healing*, London: Unwin Hynman.

Stanworth, M. (1987), *Reproductive Technologies: Gender, Motherhood and Medicine*, Cambridge: Polity.

Steiger, H. (1993), Anorexia Nervosa: is it the Syndrome or the Therapist that is Culture-and Gender-bound? *Transcultural Psychiatric Research Review*, 30, 347–58.

Strauss, A., Corbin J. (1990), *Basics of Qualitative Research: Grounded Theory Procedures and Techniques*, Newbury Park, CA: Sage.

——, J. Fagerhaugh, S., Glaser, B., Maines, D., Suczek, B., Wiener, C. (1984), *Chronic Illness and The Quality of Life*, Mosby: St Louis.

Strober, M. (1980), Personality and Symptomatological Features in Young, Nonchronic Anorexia Nervosa Patients, *Journal of Psychosomatic Research*, 21, 187–93.

Sullivan, H. S. (1954), *The Psychiatric Interview*, New York: Norton.

Swartz, L. (1987), Illness Negotiation: the Case of Eating Disorders, *Social Science and Medicine*, 24, 613–18.

Szasz, T. (1976), *The Myth of Mental Illness: Foundations of a Theory of Personal Conduct*, London: Harper and Rowe.

Szekely, E. A. (1989), From Eating Disorders to Women's Situations: Extending the Boundaries of Psychological Inquiry, *Counselling Psychology Quarterly*, 2, 167–84.

Szmukler, G., McCance, C., McCrone, L., Hunter, D. (1986), Anorexia Nervosa: a Psychiatric Case Register Study from Aberdeen, *Psychological Medicine*, 16, 49–58.

Taylor, G. J., Parker, J. D. A., Bagby, R. M., Bourke, M. P. (1996), Relationships between Alexthymia and Psychological Characteristics associated with Eating Disorders, *Journal of Psychosomatic Research*, 41, 6, 561–8.

Taylor, S., Field, D. (1993), *The Sociology of Health and Healthcare*, Oxford: Blackwell.

Thrift, N. (1994), Flies and Germs : A Geography of Knowledge. In Gregory, D. and Urry, J. (eds.) *Social Relations and Spatial Structures* (366–403) London: Macmillan.

Tolstrupp, K. (1990), Incidence and causality of Anorexia Nervosa seen in a historical perspective, *Acta Psychiatrica Scandinavica Suppl*., 361, 82, 1–6.

Toro, J., Salamero, M., Martinez, E. (1994), Assessment of Socio-Cultural Influences on the Aesthetic Body Shape Model in Anorexia, *Acta Psychiatrica Scandinavia*, 89, 147–51.

Toro, J., Cervera M., Perez, P. (1988), Body Shape, Publicity and Anorexia Nervosa. *Social Psychiatry and Psychiatric Epidemiology*, 23, 132–5.

Townsend, P., Davidson N. (1992), *Inequalities in Health: The Black Report and the Health Divide*, London: Penguin.

Turner, B. S. (1996), *The Body and Society*, (2nd ed.) London: Sage.

Twigg, J. (1983), Vegetarianism and the Meanings of Meat. In Murcott, A. (ed.) *The Sociology of Food and Eating* (18–30) Aldershot: Gower.

Ussher, J. (1991), *Women's Madness: Misogyny or Mental Illness*?, Hemel Hempstead: Harvester Wheatsheaf.

Vandereycken, W., Lowenkopf, E. (1990), Anorexia nervosa in nineteenth-century America, *Journal of Nervous and Mental Diseases*, 178, 8, 531–5.

Veblen, T. (1906), The Place of Science in Modern Civilization, American Journal of Sociology, 11, 585–609, cited in Burke, P. (2000), *A Social History of Knowledge: from Gutenberg to Diderot*, Cambridge: Polity.

Wadsworth, M. (1986), Serious Illness in Childhood and its Association with Later Life Achievement. In Wilkinson, R. (ed.) *Class and Health* (50–74), London: Tavistock.

Warde, A. (1997), *Consumption, Food and Taste*, Sage: London.

——, Heatherington, K. (1994), English households and routine food practices: a research note, *Sociological Review*, 42(4): 758–78.

Wearing, B. (1996), *Gender: The Pain and Pleasure of Difference*, Melbourne: Longman, cited in Williams, L., Germov, J. (2004), The Thin Ideal: Women, Food and Dieting. In Germov, J., Williams, L. (eds.), *A Sociology of Food and Nutrition: The Social Appetite*, (2nd ed.) Oxford University Press: Melbourne.

Webb, C. (1993), Feminist Research, Definitions, Methodology and Evaluation, *Journal of Advanced Nursing*, 18, 416–23.

Wedenoja, M. (1991) Mothers are Not to Blame: Confronting Cultural Bias in the Area of Serious Mental Illness. In Bricker-Jenkins, M., Hooyman, N. R., Gottlieb, N. (eds.) *Feminist Social Work Practice in Clinical Settings* (179–96) Thousand Oaks, CA: Sage.

Weeda-Manack, W. (1994), Female Sex-Role Conflicts and Eating Disorders. In Dolan, B., Gitzinger, I. (eds.) *Why Women: Gender Issues and Eating Disorders*, (54–78) London: Athlone.

Weitz, R. (2001), *The Sociology of Health, Illness and Healthcare*, Belmont, CA: Wadsworth.

Weston, R., Anderson, Y., Martin, T. (1998), *Loss and Bereavement: Managing Change*, Oxford: Blackwell Science.

Whitaker, A., Davies, M., Shaffer, D., Johnson, J., Abrams, S., Walsh, B. T., Kalikow, K. (1989), The Struggle to be Thin: A Survey of Anorexic and Bulimic Symptoms in a Non-referred Adolescent Population, *Psychological Medicine*, 19, 143–63.

Williams, G. (1984) The genesis of chronic illness: narrative re-construction, *Sociology of Health and Illness*, 6, 2, 175–200.

Williams, L. (2004), (ed.), *A Sociology of Food and Nutrition: The Social Appetite*, (2nd ed.) Oxford University Press: Melbourne.

——, Germov, J. (2004), The Thin Ideal: Women, Food and Dieting. In Germov, J., Williams, L. (eds.), *A Sociology of Food and Nutrition: The Social Appetite*, (2nd ed.), (337–67), Oxford University Press: Melbourne.

Wills, A., Olivieri, S. (1988), Anorexia Nervosa in Old Age, *Ageing and Mental Health,* 3, 239–45.

Wing J. K. (1980), Standardizing Clinical Diagnostic Judgements, *Australian and New Zealand Journal of Psychiatry*, 14, 17–20.

Wingate, B. A., Christie, M. J. (1978), Ego Strength and Body Image in Anorexia Nervosa, *Journal of Psychosomatic Research*, 22, 201–4.

Witz, A. (1992), *Professions and Patriarchy*, London: Routledge.

Woolgar, S. (1988) *Science: The Very Idea*: London: Tavistock.

Worrall-Thompson, A. (2003) *How to buy and cook real meat*, Little Books Ltd: London.

Wright, E. O. (1997), *Class Counts*, Cambridge: Cambridge University Press.

Wright, P., Treacher, A. (1982) (eds.) *The Problem of Medical Knowledge: Examining the Social Construction of Medicine*, Southampton: Edinburgh University Press.

Young, A. (1992), Reconstructing Rational Minds: Psychiatry and Morality in the Treatment of Post-traumatic Stress Disorder. In Lachmund, J., Stollberg, G. (eds.) *The Social Construction of Illness*, (115–24) Stuttgart: Franz Steiner Verlag.

Zelditch, M. (1962), Some Methodological Problems of Field Studies, *Amercian Journal of Sociology*, 67, 566–76.

Zola, I. K. (1973), Pathways to the Doctor: from Person to Patient, *Social Science and Medicine*, 7, 677–89.

—— (1966), Culture and Symptoms: An Analysis of Patients Presenting Complaints, *American Sociological Review*, 31, 615–30.

Index